William Franke delves into how disease and death force humanity to confront its deepest vulnerabilities in this profound exploration of pandemics in literature. Much like apocalyptic events, pandemics raise fundamental questions about the viability of human society, the fragility of life, and the structures that bind us together. These crises level all distinctions, revealing the often-ignored truths about inequality, mortality, and our shared existence. Yet amidst the despair, the text argues for hope—not as a solution to our vulnerability, but as an openness to life in all its uncertainty. This hope inspires us to transcend self-preservation, fostering solidarity and collective action toward a more meaningful life. The book illuminates the inexpressible dimensions of these world-shattering experiences through personal witness and reflection, offering a powerful meditation on the human condition.
— **Prof. Massimo Lollini**, *Professor Emeritus of Italian*, University of Oregon, USA

Pandemics and Apocalypse in World Literature is not just a scholarly survey but a constructive approach that gives itself the task to wrest possibilities of an eschatological hope from the night of apocalyptic despair. Written in the wake of the recent pandemics, the work deploys negative theology at its most creative possibility: it consists of an infinite affirmation of the unconditioned which nevertheless remains irreducibly ineffable. Franke brings together, without reducing their disparate character, the agonal traits of the end and the beginning, of despair and hope, of the abyss of the night and the first morning glow; and he shows, through rigorous exegesis of some of the very difficult texts, that perhaps the only task that is worthy today is to see the possibility of the radical, incalculable alterity that our history never ceases exposing us to. Dense, profound, thought-provoking.
— **Prof. Saitya Brata Das**, *Associate Professor*, JNU, India

William Franke's history of pandemic literature, from the ancient world to COVID, helps us understand what we are all still wondering about: what exactly happened to the us in 2020? The pandemic made us all more aware of the contingency of order, and the religious significance of this awareness, while overlooked by many, is for Franke the big take away. An eye-opener.
— **Prof. Sean J. McGrath**, *Professor*, Memorial University, Canada

William Franke's book is exceptionally important as it masterfully combines three areas of expertise: literary, anthropological, and philosophical-theological. On one hand, it offers an erudite and nearly unprecedentedly broad reconstruction of the phenomenology of the plague from its origins to the present, covering not only Western cultures but also Jewish and Chinese perspectives. On the other hand, it presents a sociological reflection on the deep-rooted causes of the plague's reemergence (today in the form of Covid-19) and its philosophical and existential implications. Saint Paul's saying, *spes contra spem (hope against hope)* is reimagined and explored within the context of apophatic theology. The reference to the Native American model of vital experience, along with Western and Eastern mysticism, underscores the depth of this approach.
— **Walter Minella**, Philosopher in Neurotheoretical Research Group, Pavia, Italy

William Franke meditates on the currently constitutive crisis of human materiality, as it manifests in the collective imbalance symptomatized by an epidemic and crashes in on every shoreline of our ecological future. In his distinctive reading of the unspeakability of our circumstance through *apophasis*, and the intensity of the crisis through *apokalypsis*, fresh insight breaks through for more spirited collective response.
— **Prof. Catherine Keller**, G.T. Cobb Professor of Constructive Theology, Drew Theological School, USA

Pandemics and Apocalypse in World Literature

Pandemics and Apocalypse rereads classical narratives of plague from the Bible (Exodus) and classical antiquity, both Greek (Homer, Thucydides, Sophocles) and Roman (Lucretius, Virgil, Ovid), through the Middle Ages (Dante, Boccaccio) and Modernity (Defoe, Manzoni, Artaud, Camus) as a basis for contemplating the significance of the recent Covid-19 pandemic. It concerns how we are to confront future pandemics and other inextricably related crises, notably those of an ecological nature. Responses to Covid-19 typically set everything on defeating this "enemy," but actually we cannot eliminate viruses without eliminating ourselves. We need to see the pandemic as revealing us to ourselves in our inherently vulnerable condition as a first step to admitting the infinite openness to one another and to our Ground—physical and metaphysical—that alone can save our world by engendering a different attitude, open and engaged, to one another and to the Earth as sources of our collective life.

William Franke is Professor of Comparative Literature at Vanderbilt University. He is currently Francesco de Dombrowski Professor in Residence at the Harvard University Center for Renaissance Studies (Villa I Tatti) in Florence, Italy, and Senior Fellow of the International Institute for Hermeneutics. He has been Research Fellow of the Alexander von Humboldt-Stiftung, Professor of Philosophy at the University of Macao, Visiting Professor of Philosophy at the University of Navarra, and Fulbright Distinguished Chair in Intercultural Theology and the Study of Religions at the University of Salzburg. His books include *On What Cannot Be Said* (2007); *Poetry and Apocalypse* (2009); *Dante and the Sense of Transgression* (2013); *A Philosophy of the Unsayable* (2014); *The Revelation of Imagination* (2015); *Secular Scriptures* (2016); *A Theology of Literature* (2018); *The Universality of What Is Not* (2020); *The Divine Vision of Dante's* Paradiso (2021); *The* Vita Nuova *and the New Testament* (2021); *Dante's* Paradiso *and the Theological Origins of Modern* Thought (2021); *Dantologies* (2024); *Don Quixote and the Quest for the Absolute in Literature* (2024); and others.

Routledge Focus on Literature

Essays on The Glass Menagerie
Truth in the Pleasant Disguise of Illusion
Tania Chakravertty

Margaret Wise Brown's Experimental Art
The Modernist Picture Book
Julia Pond

Tolkien and the Kalevala
Jyrki Korpua

Elevating Humanity via Africana Womanism
Clenora Hudson (Weems)

Reading Modernity, Modernism and Religion Today
Spinoza and Van Gogh
Patrick Grant

The Sagas of Icelanders
An Introduction to All Forty Sagas with Summaries
Annette Lassen

Pandemics and Apocalypse in World Literature
The Hope for Planetary Salvation
William Franke

Reading Kazuo Ishiguro's *Never Let Me Go*
The Alternative Dystopian Imagination
Eva Pelayo Sañudo

For more information about this series, please visit: www.routledge.com/Routledge-Focus-on-Literature/book-series/RFLT

Pandemics and Apocalypse in World Literature
The Hope for Planetary Salvation

William Franke

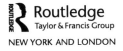

NEW YORK AND LONDON

First published 2025
by Routledge
605 Third Avenue, New York, NY 10158

and by Routledge
4 Park Square, Milton Park, Abingdon, Oxon, OX14 4RN

Routledge is an imprint of the Taylor & Francis Group, an informa business

© 2025 William Franke

The right of William Franke to be identified as author of this work has been asserted in accordance with sections 77 and 78 of the Copyright, Designs and Patents Act 1988.

All rights reserved. No part of this book may be reprinted or reproduced or utilised in any form or by any electronic, mechanical, or other means, now known or hereafter invented, including photocopying and recording, or in any information storage or retrieval system, without permission in writing from the publishers.

Trademark notice: Product or corporate names may be trademarks or registered trademarks, and are used only for identification and explanation without intent to infringe.

ISBN: 978-1-032-89585-7 (hbk)
ISBN: 978-1-032-90027-8 (pbk)
ISBN: 978-1-003-54583-5 (ebk)

DOI: 10.4324/9781003545835

Typeset in Times New Roman
by SPi Technologies India Pvt Ltd (Straive)

Contents

List of Illustrations   x

1 Prologue and Acknowledgments   1

PART I
Plague Literature   7

2 The Engendering of Hope from Human Helplessness   9

3 Myth, History, Fiction, and the Limits of Representation   20

4 The Mystery of the Supernatural at the Limit of Naturalism   25

5 From Ambiguity of Causes to Moral Certitude through Existential Conversion   30

6 Securing Control versus Acknowledging Grace and Vulnerability   36

7 Hope in a Negative Theological and Apocalyptic-Fictive Register of Wholeness   40

8 Theology of Hope as Negative Theology—Moltmann and Bloch   48

9 Partial Action Combined with Hope in Wholeness   51

10 Othering Hope: Postmodern, Extra-European, and Indigenous Perspectives ... 53

11 The Vision of the Whole versus Parceled Perception ... 59

PART II
Political Ecology ... 61

12 The Web of Connections: Integral Ecology, Culture, and Society ... 63

13 Pandemics and Environmental Apocalypse: Their Common Causes ... 68

14 Progressive versus Apocalyptic Perspectives on Pandemics ... 72

15 Hope in Civil Society between Private and Public ... 77

16 From Social to Cosmic Consciousness: Latour's Apocalyptic Reading of the Coronavirus Crisis ... 79

17 Relativizing Scientific "Truth" ... 82

18 Truth and Transcendence versus Technique ... 85

19 Negative Theology of the Earth According to Bruno Latour ... 87

PART III
Apocalyptic Hope ... 91

20 Eschatology, Incarnation, Kenosis ... 93

21 Indigenous Salvation as Guide ... 99

22 From "Theology of Hope" to "Theology of the Earth" ... 101

23 Science, Faith, and Social Belief—Not Strictly Separable ... 104

24	Control and Excess in Dissembling the Unspeakable	107
25	Parallel Perspectives and the Novel	111
26	A Semiotic Model of Contagion—Viral Informatics	113
27	Hoping against Hope: From Reason to Religion, or Spiritualizing Rationality	115
28	Conclusion: Hope-Fail Enactment of Eternity	119
29	Coda: Plague and War	123
30	Appendix: Abstracts of Selected Plague Narratives in Literature, Classical to Modern	127
	Bibliography	*135*
	Index	*143*

Illustrations

2.1	"Egyptian Plague of Boils," Toggenburg Bible, 1411	14
2.2	"Triumph of Death," Pieter Brueghel, 1562	18
5.1	"Franciscan monks treating victims of the plague," Jacopo Oddi (d. 1474)	32
7.1	"Torture and execution of 'anointers' in 1630 Milanese plague," Anon.	42
7.2	"Triumph of Death," unknown master, Palazzo Abbatellis, Palermo, 1446	44
27.1	"Roman Plague Allegory," Jules Elie Delauney, 1869	118
29.1	"Gods Descending to Battle," John Flaxman's *Iliad,* 1795	126

"Hope" is the thing with feathers -
That perches in the soul -
And sings the tune without the words -
And never stops - at all -

              Emily Dickinson

Laudato si', mi' Signore,
per sora nostra matre Terra,
la quale ne sustenta e governa,
e produce diversi frutti con coloriti fiori et herba ...

Laudato si', mi' Signore,
per sora nostra Morte corporale,
da la quale nullu homo vivente po' skappare ...

           Saint Francis of Assisi

(Be praised, my Lord,
for our sister Mother Earth,
who sustains and governs us
and produces diverse fruits with colored flowers and grass ...

Be praised, my Lord,
for our sister corporeal Death,
from whom no living man can escape ...)

1 Prologue and Acknowledgments

During confinement for the Covid-19 pandemic, many of us were moved to look back to source texts in classical literature in search of historical perspectives and precedents that might offer guidance as to how such epidemic outbreaks had been confronted in the past. I, too, organized my seminar at Vanderbilt University (Nashville, Tennessee) in spring semester 2021 around the theme: "Pandemic and Apocalypse in World Literature," taking on a topic with which we were all, by force of circumstances, struggling mightily. As is my wont, I wrote out my thoughts in order to prepare for my lectures, and these preparations provided me with the core material for this book.

However, this material came to be shaped into a continuous argument and was composed into the form of a book thanks only to a more specific occasion, namely, an invitation to deliver a keynote address for a transdisciplinary, international conference titled "Processing the Pandemic III: Hope." The conference was of a curiously hybrid nature: it was sponsored jointly by the Centre for the Study of the Renaissance at the University of Warwick, England, and the Center for Renaissance Studies, coupled with the D'Arcy McNickle Center for American Indian and Indigenous Studies, at the Newberry Library, Chicago, Illinois. I found intriguing the idea of exploring how Renaissance Studies and Indigenous Studies might be made to meet up and dance together, and so I buried scholarly scruples and plucked up courage to accept the invitation and take on this challenge.

This "transdisciplinary symposium around the theme of hope," as stated in the Call for Papers, was to be the third event in a trilogy, following a "first in-person symposium on 'Loss' at the Newberry Library in April 2022 and an ongoing series of virtual seminars." Held physically at the University of Warwick on April 13–14, 2023, this further in-person conference on the topic unfolding in several phases was billed as "the final event in the series" and as "the final phase of Processing the Pandemic: a multi-year series of seminars and symposia that explore how the

DOI: 10.4324/9781003545835-1

experiences of the past may guide society's emotional and social responses to the COVID-19 pandemic."[1]

As the time for the conference drew near and the titles of the talks were being finalized, I received a message from the organizing committee that they were holding up publication of the conference program because of some concerns that had arisen around the title I had submitted for my lecture. This title originally was: "Pandemics and Apocalypse in World Literature and Indigenous Salvation." After a few rounds of politely veiled hints and innuendos, it became clear to me what the problem was. It was possible to hear the words "Indigenous Salvation" as a reprise of Christian colonial missionary rhetoric.

Of course, the committee knew, as they assured me, that this way of understanding the terms of my title was not what I intended, but it was feared nevertheless that some members of the prospective audience, including especially its online extension on both sides of the Atlantic, might hear it that way. I could see their point. I had not been thinking of that. By the phrase "Indigenous Salvation" I had intended rather to indicate the potential for us to learn about spiritual health and ecological well-being from Indigenous communities and from the traditions and attitudes they might model vis-à-vis pandemics.

On reflection, it occurred to me that this phrase had seemed resonantly right precisely *because* there was a history behind it, not one that I had had present to mind, but a history with an opaque density that was still actively operating and that concealed much work still to be done. I realized through this exchange that I had unconsciously, yet quite purposefully, undertaken to reverse a certain historical discourse on "Indigenous Salvation," of which, after all, I had been well-aware from long before beginning my project. I was looking to the Indigenous to become our guides indicating the way to salvation rather than the ones needing to be saved. I had been aiming, albeit "through a glass darkly," to reconceive and reinvest this language with a new sense opposite to what it had meant in historical colonialist discourse, the echo of which in my title had now become unmistakable to me.

Even without having fully realized it, my hope was to relaunch the idea of "salvation" (taken to its Latin roots as *salus*, health) with a wholly different spin and with an ear turned toward what Indigenous cultures might have to say about healthily harmonizing with one's environment in respect and reverence for the Earth. I thought that by this means I could make a vital, even if theoretical and speculative, contribution to fostering "open and transformative conversations," as the statement outlining the conference's purposes proposed. Although reluctantly, I accepted the

---

1 Citations from the CFP: Newberry Library | Processing the Pandemic III: Hope. Accessed 3-20-2023.

committee's erasure of the words "Indigenous Salvation" from my title. The thrust of my argument remained still intact since it centered not so directly on the idea of salvation as on *hope*, following the stated topic and promptings from the organizer who had corresponded with me at the time of my invitation and had determined with me the precise subject of my lecture.

With some discussion indebted also to my wife, Béatrice Machet, the translator of numerous contemporary Native American poets into French, I proposed to substitute for "salvation" the term "survivance," which I had already introduced into the paper thanks to some direct personal contact and exchange with Anishinaabe author Gerald Vizenor. Vizenor had visited France earlier in the year and had given a talk that Béatrice (with my collaboration) had translated simultaneously. The occasion had given me the opportunity for extensive exchange with Vizenor in public and in private. Together we discovered his notion of "survivance," or using means of resistance that are non-oppositional and rely more on irony, to be a strategy consonant with what I think through and enact in the terms of a negative theology plied as a form of praxis. As oblique, negative forms of verbal acting, these strategies bear an affinity to kenotic self-emptying, or even to Daoist "non-action," *wu wei*. However, my proposed substitution of "survivance" for "salvation" did not convince the committee either. They preferred simply to leave reference to the Indigenous out of my title. Other speakers were going to be addressing that part of the program, and it would best be left to them.

There was also an understandable concern expressed by a committee member that we should avoid generalizing about Indigenous cultures. My reply was that my purpose was not to discuss in any detailed and differentiated way particular Indigenous cultures. I had not been asked to do that. In fact, I had been invited specifically to represent the Medieval and Early Modern wing of the conference and been told that there would be someone else to speak for the Indigenous component. But the conference Call for Papers, nevertheless, named Native American and Indigenous Studies first among the humanities disciplines it intended to engage. This made sense, given the co-sponsorship of the conference by the D'Arcy McNickle Center for American Indian and Indigenous Studies. Consequently, I wished to indicate an openness for dialogue with Indigenous and Native American cultures on this topic. Simply to ignore what was such an important, equally weighted component of the conference might also run a risk of repeating certain hurtful patterns of the past. I planned to foster such dialogue by my kind of speculative thinking, moving between the disciplines especially of philosophy and theology and of literary and cultural criticism.

The synthesis that I present in what follows and that I had conceived already in preparation for the conference, entails what I call "negative theology," or thinking that is oriented and normed by an ineffable, inconceivable absolute. Theology, when qualified as *negative*, disowns or undoes even itself as a *logos* or science of *theos* by admitting that it cannot know exactly what its designated subject, "God," is or means (God only knows). We know only what God is *not*. Such an orientation entails, therefore, as constitutive of negative theology, a recursive, self-critical reflection on its own limits in relation to a supposed or imaginable Ground that it cannot think (whether or not such a ground actually "exists").

Such negative theological reflection resets more than just theology. Not only God but everything is unknowable in its absoluteness. We know only our own *relation* to every Other and realizing this changes our relation to everything. Such reflection can be extended, furthermore, far beyond the epistemological or ontological domains to embrace consequences for ethics and action and passion. Negative theological reflection, as I construe and practice it, leads to an awareness of the totally relational nature of our being and to acceptance of our unsurpassable vulnerability to others. This vulnerability shows up as an ineluctable interdependence of all on one another, which is ever more acutely felt in a world of shrinking resources, a world that is becoming more and more crowded. Relating to the other person in their inexhaustible mystery and transcendence reveals to us an infinite dimension of our openness to alterity and our beholdenness to one another. Such a dimension can be poetically concretized and pragmatically schematized as an, at least imaginable, relation to an unthinkably absolute Other, or to an ultimate alterity, imagined, for instance, as the Earth, on which our own being together with that of every other living being depends in order to be at all.

There is thus also a positive aspect, a constructive and creative side, to the critical, self-limiting, and self-exposing type of thinking that I model on negative theology. Such thinking is plied here to trace out how Jürgen Moltmann's Theology of Hope, building on the utopian philosophical reflections of Ernst Bloch, can be made to evolve into a Theology of the Earth in the wake of Bruno Latour's late, ecologically engaged philosophy. Although we lose in technical mastery over our designated subject matter, we gain infinitely more in positive resonance and relatedness beyond the limits of our own endemic self-enclosure.

My aim was, and is, to suggest where I see some openings for dialogue between traditions based on what they do not—and perhaps cannot—say more than on any of their articulated teachings and express doctrines. Concerning Indigenous cultures, the potential is immense for enabling us to re-inherit terms like "salvation" and understand them in previously undreamt-of ways. Reflection on and around such a term and its substitutes or transforms, like "survivance," can open pathways to the uncannily revealing synergisms that are possible here. Indigenous perspectives open upon the dimension of the planetary. All these terms indicate mighty challenges that faced a symposium of the unusually, not to say awkwardly, hybrid type that had been planned.

The essay and the book it has become largely exceed the parameters of the conference alluded to here as its originating occasion. Yet this motivating matrix remains central for orienting the entire reflection and so is recalled here and brought forward as its informing context. This permits a rooting of my re-thinking of classical through modern traditions of thought on pandemics in current critical discussion. Particularly the issues and sensitivities emerging around Indigenous cultures and our relation to the Earth have spawned new horizons to be explored.

Unfolding in a continuous flow of interconnected concepts, the book is poetic as much as analytic in form. A progression of predominant motifs permits successive chapters to be grouped into broadly themed parts. However, each chapter and part, in myriad ways, remains open and connected to every other. They reciprocally reflect on one another in a scintillating dynamic. This organization highlights literature's potential to serve not only as a method of argument but also as a means of revelation which culminates in apocalypse. Linearity is made to work multilaterally to transcend itself into *totum simul* vision.

I thank the organizing committee (particularly Bryan Brazeau, Christopher Fletcher, and Rose Miron) for their invitation and engagement with me on this topic, as well as all participants for their responses and for the many enlightening exchanges we had at and after the conference in Warwick. I acknowledge equally the stimulating exchange with Vanderbilt students during the coronavirus crisis and our course on this topic, which, regrettably but unavoidably, could take place only online and at a distance (from the south of France, in my case). This circumstance made us all the more acutely and concretely aware of how the pandemic was reorganizing our lives.

Translations from foreign language texts, unless otherwise attributed, are my own. Bible quotations follow the Authorized King James Version (1611) corrected, where necessary, by the Greek New Testament and the Vulgate.

William Franke
Villa La Réunion,
Carcès, Var (Provence)
France

Part I
Plague Literature

2 The Engendering of Hope from Human Helplessness

The Covid-19 (SARS-CoV-2) pandemic has spread far beyond the parameters of medical science and public health. It has pushed our societies and their systems of symbolization to new limits and thresholds. The full consequences will emerge only gradually over the course of ensuing years. The following reflections formulate some preliminary hypotheses concerning this generalized crisis that has become a human tragedy in numerous and diverse registers: psychological, social, and cultural, as well as in its more obvious medical and economic repercussions. More specifically, these reflections reformulate and reanimate certain perennial insights, drawn especially from history and literature, as saving and revelatory for our own time. The pandemic strikes differently at different levels of society and across distant regions around the world. It has made burning questions regarding equality and justice in society and the world all the more flagrant.

One terrifying, yet potentially salutary and unexpected, effect, in the midst of the mayhem, has been to reveal us to ourselves. *Hope* has to begin with and center on this augmented self-awareness. This is our initial point of departure. We are forced to face hard truths that, otherwise, it is all too tempting to look away from and persist in denying. Such facing-up realizes a cathartic purpose that pandemics since antiquity have constantly served. Plagues effect a kind of purge. The revelation forced on us by pandemics is apocalyptic, furthermore, in that its disclosure reaches all the way to the end of our world. For individuals, this means to death, which alone enables us to see—and thence to reconceive and appropriate—our lives whole.

In this regard, the current pandemic (which has spilled over into ongoing crises) is not without precedents just as piercing in their revelatory power as they are harrowing in their effects on their victims. Numerous previous passes in human history, with its recurring epidemics, have brought about similar comeuppances. Taken together, they call for comparison—even though there is also something final or "apocalyptic" about each such realization for the individuals involved in every unique

DOI: 10.4324/9781003545835-3

instance of pandemic. Beyond these personal, pathetic perspectives, there is also a potential for a general apocalyptic disclosure of the alpha and omega, a visionary seeing of things whole.

The realization and even revelation provoked by pandemics is, in any case, mediated by imagination, which means also by emotion. Hence the importance of *literature* for "processing" pandemics. Human and cultural mediation is at work in news reporting and chronicling, as well as in commentary and investigative journalism. But it is present all the more penetratingly in the more deeply reflective and deliberately imaginative expressions or representations found in literature. A chief purpose of mine in addressing this topic is to resource outstanding testimonies in literary works concerning historical or fictive plagues and pandemics—especially visionary works of recognized genius. Revisiting these classics stimulates reflection turned finally toward our own present dilemmas in the current crisis.

I say "current" because, even though the Covid-19 pandemic has now been declared to be at an end in almost all Western countries, we nevertheless live in an ongoing condition of crisis and trauma that the COronaVIrusDisease-2019 pandemic triggered in dramatic ways and that is not going away. The enormity of this upheaval is felt relative to our own recent direct experience, but it is not unique. The broader horizon of human history across millennia presents the repeated spectacle of periodic catastrophes not less distressing than all that we have experienced.

Plague descriptions abound in literature from the Bible (Exodus) and classical antiquity, both Greek (Homer, Sophocles, Thucydides) and Latin (Lucretius, Virgil, Ovid), through the Middle Ages (Dante, Boccaccio) and the early modern period (Daniel Defoe), passing on to Italian Romanticism (Alessandro Manzoni) and French surrealism (Antonin Artaud) and existentialism (Albert Camus). Narratives by all these authors reflect on the sobering experience of being forced by plague-provoked catastrophes to face certain complacency-shattering truths about life and death that we otherwise inevitably contrive to fool ourselves about and elude. In subtly variegated ways, each pandemic episode, as commemorated in literature, holds up a mirror to our present predicament and its quandaries. I am not the first to try and sift the significance of this literary archive. But my assessment, for all its grounding in tradition, is a unique response and not like what others are saying on the subject.

Samuel Weber offers critical interpretations of mostly the same roster of classic texts of Western tradition, with some significant variations, yet he provides virtually no treatment of the Latin classics (Lucretius being cited only in his book's epigraph) or of Manzoni or Wright. He emphasizes how the narration of plague serves to reveal as "preexisting conditions" what are fundamental, structural flaws conditioning society.

The Engendering of Hope from Human Helplessness   11

They are already in place and festering long before the manifest outbreaks of the disease.[1]

For Judith Butler, this revelation, at least as realized by the Covid-19 pandemic, is a disclosure of our lack of a "common world" and, at the same time, of our interconnectedness in dependency on common resources without borders. Even our bodies can hardly be kept separate and discreet from one another. Butler draws on Maurice Merleau-Ponty's phenomenological descriptions of the intertwining of our lives and bodies with those of others in a common world. Such intertwining (which Merleau-Ponty often figures as "chiasmus," evoking the infinite open-endedness of the Greek letter X, with its sprawling open arms) has usually remained latent and unrealized but is now startlingly revealed to us by the pandemic. Butler draws also on Max Scheler's analysis of the "phenomenon of the tragic" in order to interrogate the "sense of the world." She underscores "the destruction of value" (notably the value of lives and of the earth), which defines the tragic for Scheler, as unequally borne by some.[2]

For Butler, "the structure of the world can be understood only through a radical epistemic dislocation. The world was not as one thought it was ..." (68). Applying a phenomenology of the tragic, Butler cogently observes that a pandemic is the type of event that ruptures our current notion of the world and its possibilities as bound within a certain "horizon" and reopens the world to infinity. "Whatever limit is imposed by the notion of a horizon has to be rethought in terms of the infinity that, as it were, runs through and exceeds it" (69). In my understanding, breaking the world open again to the Infinite is the salutary function of the pandemic that produces unsuspected possibilities of hope for reconceiving the world anew.

The commonality of our world has remained largely concealed, among other reasons, because globalization fragments society along lines of class and capital as determinants of different, parallel worlds. Slavoj Žižek, in another recent, high-profile treatment of the subject, sees the pandemic as revealing the necessity of forging a new form of "communism" after the motto "We're all in the same boat now." However, he puts us on guard against drawing any conclusions as to the sense or meaning of the pandemic as a kind of moral of the story:

> However, we should resist the temptation to treat the ongoing epidemic as something that has a deeper meaning: the cruel but just punishment of humanity for the ruthless exploitation of other forms

---

1 Samuel Weber, *Preexisting Conditions: Recounting the Plague* (New York: Zone Books, 2022).
2 Judith Butler, *What World Is This? A Pandemic Phenomenology* (New York: Columbia University Press, 2022), 19–45.

of life on earth. If we search for such a hidden message, we remain premodern: we treat our universe as a partner in communication. Even if our very survival is threatened, there is something reassuring in the fact that we are punished, the universe (or even Somebody-out-there) is engaging with *us*. We matter in some profound way. The really difficult thing to accept is the fact that the ongoing epidemic is a result of natural contingency at its purest, that it just happened and hides no deeper meaning.[3]

Žižek warns against moralizing readings, but he misses, or at least minimizes, the more profound existential and negative theological meaning that the classic narratives, as well as some popular treatments of plague, subtly suggest. This is a meaning traversed by meaninglessness, but it is not attained by abjuring and placing an interdiction on all meaning whatsoever. Our chosen texts are open fields for the work of sifting, forging, and deconstructing meanings, as well as for opening them and ourselves to our beholdenness to one another.

Indeed, we are all in the same boat at the level of existence that matters most. Yet Žižek's worry about falling into premodern patterns of thought perhaps causes him to remain stuck in the modern prejudice that underwrites a certain myth of progress by surpassing the theological, metaphysical illusion of "Somebody-out-there." In this posture, he falls short of articulating what I consider to be a fully *post*modern perspective—one in which certain *pre*modern views can once again make sense and shed light on perennial aspects of our contemporary predicament. Such views enable us to break free from constricting modern dogmas. This is the task that I take up with a vision of world literature different from Weber's (who, in the name of "modesty," abjures hope for "salvation," 194–95; cf. 135) and with a social agenda and cultural politics different from Butler's. In my vision, poetic truth and religious revelation are mutually enabling experiences that allow us also to see a deeper sense in traditional texts and to understand our world more comprehensively—beyond artificial periodizations and Žižek's presumed surpassing of our premodern past.

Lawrence Wright's novel *The End of October* (2020) was researched and written shortly before the outbreak of Covid-19 but prophetically anticipates many of its most horrific and hallucinatory features. Wright's work of contemporary fiction brings my historical survey of selected samples from world literature up to date near to our own time on the eve of a recent outbreak of pandemic and the global panic it let loose upon the world. A best-selling thriller, Wright's novel opens our topic conspicuously to the archives of popular culture, which since the Middle Ages has

---

3 Slavoj Žižek, *Pandemic: COVID-19 Shakes the World* (Cambridge: Polity Press, 2020), 14. Cf. 103–104.

The Engendering of Hope from Human Helplessness

left riveting testimonies about the traumatic experience of pandemics, often in an apocalyptic perspective.[4]

These historical and/or fictionalized accounts of literal plagues imaging literal death by disease, however, are not the whole story or the only approach. There are also moral or spiritual contagions, "plagues" in a metaphorical and/or allegorical sense, infecting the whole human race that have been powerfully represented in literature throughout the ages. These non-biological "pandemics" may even have been revealed and realized for the first time in their full purport only *through* literature. The notion of pandemic disease works apocalyptically in our cultural imaginary and has everything to do with how we respond to pandemics concretely. Accordingly, these moral or metaphorical plagues can be every bit as consequential as the literal ones.

Sometimes such metaphorical pandemic narratives have been able to penetrate and determine the underlying symbolic system of whole cultures. A prime example is the theological myth of the Fall of Man represented most influentially by Saint Augustine as a kind of disease transmitted to all sexually. Adam's Fall into sin becomes manifest in every one of his descendants from the moment of their birth.[5] A universal state of congenital illness and susceptibility to moral degeneration is expressed in the newborn babe's wailing as it gasps for its first breaths of air in the external, postnatal world. Sin is manifest a little later in the baby's willfully manipulative crying to make others obey its wishes. Augustine also observes infants' wishing to deprive other babies as potential rivals for the maternal breast.[6] He interprets this as proof of an innate, original state of non-innocence. He attributes it to a kind of moral disease contracted at conception overshadowed by the sin of concupiscence in the sexual act.

At the biblical source behind Augustine's interpretation stands Saint Paul's understanding of the Fall from Edenic health and happiness. Paul's Epistle to the Romans, Chapter 5, arguably reads the sin of Adam and Eve in Genesis 3 as the original pandemic, the pandemic of all pandemics. This "original" sin becomes a kind of hereditary disease or disablement that renders the entire human race morally infirm: "as by one man sin entered into the world, and death by sin; and so death passed upon all men, for that all have sinned" (Romans 5:12). Adam's—and even more originally Eve's—sin becomes the Pandora's box out which every sort of ill is released into the world. Adam's and Eve's so-called Original Sin is

---

4 See the Newberry Library's site: Learning from Premodern Plagues – Digital Collections for the Classroom (newberry.org). Accessed 4-4-2023.

5 Most important here are Augustine's anti-Pelagian writings, particularly *De gratia Christi et de peccato originali* II, 40.45. CSEL (*Corpus Scriptorum Ecclesiasticorum Latinorum*) 42, 202 [23–25], *Patrologiae cursus Completus: Series Latina*, ed. J. P. Minge (Paris: Migne, 1844–1864) 44, 407. Cf. *De civitate Dei* XIV, 11–16.

6 Augustine, *Confessions*, Book I, vii, 11.

held to infect the will with a kind of corruption to which humankind ever after is heir. This state of fallenness is like a disease to be remedied only by the advent of Christ, who redeems us from Adam's sin through the Cross (Romans 7). Milton's elaboration of these themes in *Paradise Lost* takes them to certain sublime heights of literary expression and artifice.

In a literary vein, the physical and the moral or spiritual aspects of plagues tend to be indissoluble. Plagues are signs of moral corruption or of a religious stain, an offense against the gods. This is the case in the Bible, for example, in the ten plagues cast on Egypt, targeting Pharaoh, his army, and his people, in the Book of Exodus (Illustration 2.1). It is clearly the case again in classical epic (at the beginning of the *Iliad*) and in ancient tragedy, signally in Sophocles's *Oedipus Rex* and in Seneca's *Oedipus*, a first-century CE apocalyptic remake of Sophocles's drama. That plagues are the direct consequence of human moral outrages or sin is a common motif also in folklore, where the offended parties are sometimes fairies responsible for regulating natural cycles.[7] Moral or spiritual disorder is manifest as physical corruption causing death and disease. Sickness figures as rampant across the land and as pervasive also in the

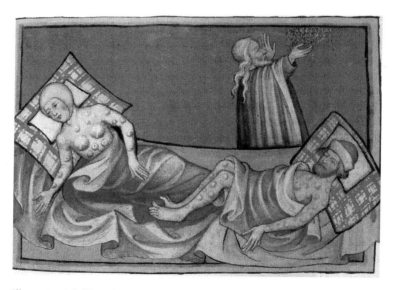

Illustration 2.1 "Egyptian Plague of Boils," Toggenburg Bible, 1411.

7 See, for instance, Theodor Storm, "Märchen von der Regentrüde," *Leipziger illustrierte Zeitung*, July 30, 1863, in Theodor Storm, *Sämtliche Werke in vier Bänden*, ed. Peter Goldhammer (Berlin: Aufbau, 1978).

social realm throughout the kingdom, up and down its hierarchized echelons, from pauper to king.

Such allegorical applications of the image of plague and pandemic as correlates to, or visible expressions of, moral disorder are legion. The sources just mentioned consistently interpret real pandemic disease as signs of some kind of primal transgression or crime—incest and patricide in the case of King Oedipus. In the *Iliad*, an offense against a priest of Apollo named Chryses, whose daughter Chryseis is being held captive by Agamemnon, stands at the source of the plague (*loimos*–λοιμός) that through the agency of the archer god slaughters the Greeks by their ships in their camp even more redoubtably, more miserably and ingloriously, than do their human foes on the battle fields before the city gates of Troy.

These examples suggest how plague and pandemic may be evoked symbolically wherever the aim is to signify a hidden moral contagion or pervasive social corruption, or even just a crime by an individual who is responsible for contaminating a collectivity. Plague can become a general symbolic indicator of whatever is ill about humanity.

Primo Levi is one of a number of authors who invite us to view pandemic disease allegorically through the lens of the Nazi death camps. Social maladies of all sorts have a way of becoming infectious and spreading by dint of the inherently imitative and associate nature of social intercourse. Epidemic disease turns up as an obvious and practically ubiquitous symbol for whatever "plagues" human society. Albert Camus's *The Plague* (*La peste*, 1947) elaborates the pestilence besieging Algerian Oran as an allegory of the Nazis' death-dealing stranglehold on Europe. This allegorical intent is avowed expressly by Camus in his notebooks and has remained central to criticism of the novel ever since.[8]

But plague, in any case, alludes to something that surpasses all humanly ascertainable reality. The idea of plague as retribution from heaven lurks near and looms large over these accounts, even when such an idea is openly contested or subjected to ridicule. Camus captures the derisive spirit in which superstitious notions about the plague's causes are mocked even by those being devastated by forces beyond their control. Indeed, the mocking "humanists" who refuse supernatural explanations are derided in turn by the facts:

> Our fellow citizens in this regard were like everyone else, they were thinking of themselves, or in other words they were humanists: they did not believe in divine scourges. The scourge is not within the reach of man; therefore, one says it is unreal, a bad dream that will pass. But it does not always pass, and from bad dream to bad dream it is humans

---

8 Albert Camus, *Carnets: Janvier 1942-Mars 1951*, vol. 2 (Paris: Gallimard, 1964), xx, trans. Justin O'Brien as *Notebooks: 1942-1951* (New York: Knopf, 1966).

who pass, and humanists in the first place because they did not take precautions. Our fellow citizens were not more guilty than others; they forgot to be modest, that's all, and they thought that all could still be possible for them, which presupposed that scourges are impossible.

Nos concitoyens à cet égard étaient comme tout le monde, ils pensaient à eux-mêmes, autrement dit ils étaient humanistes : ils ne croyaient pas aux fléaux. Le fléau n'est pas à la mesure de l'homme, on se dit donc que le fléau est irréel, c'est un mauvais rêve qui va passer. Mais il ne passe pas toujours et, de mauvais rêve en mauvais rêve, ce sont les hommes qui passent, et les humanistes, en premier lieu, parce qu'ils n'ont pas pris leurs précautions. Nos concitoyens n'étaient pas plus coupables que d'autres, ils oubliaient d'être modestes, voilà tout, et ils pensaient que tout était encore possible pour eux, ce qui supposait que les fléaux étaient impossibles.[9]

Plague, as a scourge from heaven, is deemed "impossible" because we have no hope of dealing with it by any human means. If we cannot combat and overcome it, it cannot exist. This is typical "humanist" reasoning, as Camus construes it. Is there, then, a different kind of hope in what is not within our own means and methods, a hope that breaks us open beyond ourselves into relation with something other and absolute, something perhaps divine or, in any case, real beyond our control and comprehension? Is this other sort of relatedness beyond our own human self-relatedness the lesson that humanity is repeatedly taught and has had to learn over and over from the agonizing experience of pandemics, most recently the Covid-19 crisis? Is this infinite openness to the Other not what we need to learn also in order to avert war with one another, which is tearing our world apart, as well as to escape ecological injustice toward other living species that results finally in the destruction of Earth itself?

What is "impossible" for Camus's modern humanists, with their faith in human progress, becomes paramount from a postmodern viewpoint peering beyond the human to the posthuman and beyond the modern project of unlimited progress. Jacques Derrida (1930–2004), another declared atheist in the French philosophical tradition scarcely a generation after Camus (1913–60), would come to focus precisely on *the impossible* as what most needs to be thought.[10] What is impossible within our humanly constructed order and system of thought challenges us to exceed

9 Albert Camus, *La peste* (Paris: Gallimard, 1947), 40–41.
10 "L'impossible" is a pervasive theme throughout Derrida's later works, for example, *Sauf le nom*, *Passions*, and *Khôra*. It is thematized directly in "Non pas l'utopie, l'im-possible," in *Papier Machine* (Paris: Galilée, 2001). Derrida's ethics of the impossible are treated in brief compass by François Raffoul, "Derrida et l'éthique de l'im-possible," *Revue de métaphysique et de morale* 53/1 (2007): 73–88.

ourselves and to confront something radically and irreducibly *Other*. Derrida understood this challenge as a kind of summons or calling with apocalyptic undertones and overtones.[11] This postmodern turn, brought about by Derrida and company, came in the wake of Martin Heidegger's critique and surpassing of humanism ("Letter on Humanism," 1946) and its ethos of technological domination of the planet understood as the legacy of metaphysics—which Heidegger's thinking aimed to overcome.[12]

Plague devastates humans beyond their capacity to control or escape it. This is why it has always been interpreted, at least by some of those seized in its grip, as a judgment from God. Without presupposing any determinate theology, I want to emphasize that pandemics force us to confront an absolute reality, or an absoluteness of the real, that transcends human manipulation and management. Plague reminds us of our impotence and wakes us up to recognition of what utterly surpasses our capacity to resist. Particularly plague's inseparable specter, death, must be recognized as an unnegotiable limit that leaves humans powerless, hard as that is for us to accept. But also, no matter how healthily we strive to live, we are all subject to sudden destructive disease striking us down unexpectedly. This insurmountable vulnerability, I submit, is the most universal and far-reaching significance of plague or pandemic that can be inferred from the works of many of our most clairvoyant authors across the ages.

It is telling that from ancient and medieval authors like Homer and Boccaccio to Defoe and modern novelists, plague has been consistently interpreted as a scourge for human waywardness and sin. The terrible specter of the Black Death rearing its ugly visage is treated in all imaginable manners as a terrifying punishment ordained from above—from heaven. The confrontation with a superior power that annihilates humans finally in death is brought on the scene as a constant threat that comes to consciousness whenever and wherever pestilence strikes (Illustration 2.2).

This is the first and most obvious way in which pandemics evoke a theological dimension reaching to the Infinite beyond human grasp. We face our own annihilation by what is an absolute power lording it over us and crushing us. This confrontation with annihilation constitutes the ground for opening to a dimension of ultimacy, a dimension that invites theological and specifically apocalyptic interpretation—or at least negative theological speculation. Whether or not we can put any positive description of divinity on it, we find ourselves faced with an unconditional absolute to

---

11 Derrida, "No apocalypse, not now: à toute vitesse, sept missives, sept missiles," *Les Cahiers du GRIF*, 41–42 (1989), L'imaginaire du nucléaire, 79-8, trans. Catherine Porter and Philip Lewis as "No Apocalypse, Not Now (Full Speed Ahead, Seven Missiles, Seven Missives), *Diacritics* 14/2, Nuclear Criticism (1984): 20–31.

12 Martin Heidegger, *Über den Humanismus* (Frankfurt am Main: Klostermann, 1949), translated as "Letter on Humanism," in Martin Heidegger, *Basic Works*, ed. David Farrell Krell (New York: Harper & Row, 1977), 190–242.

18 *Pandemics and Apocalypse in World Literature*

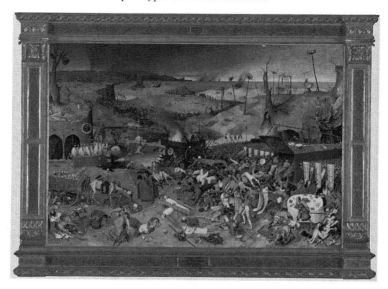

Illustration 2.2 "Triumph of Death," Pieter Brueghel, 1562.

which we are subjected, even abjectly, as it annihilates our very being in the world.

The book in hand aims to disclose a "theological" meaning as intrinsic to the idea of plague or pandemic, but not in a fatalistic sense. Instead, theology—or more exactly *negative theology*—entails essentially recognition of a reality beyond our own ordering and management, reality as other to the systems we make. This Other is the source of the hope I consider to be genuinely hopeful against our delusion of mastering everything through our technologies—our vaccinations, quarantines, border controls, carrier tests, contact tracings, curfews, confinements, protective masks, and the rest. All these technical measures can work as alibis and ersatz offerings that engender a falsely comforting kind of illusory hope, even a temptation of an escapist nature, and result in a failure to face the fundamental problem of our relation to the real. We fail to recognize any reality greater than us commanding us from beyond our control.

There is always something absurd about death, even when it arrives as naturally as can be. Camus, for one, contemplates and rebels against this absurdity—most explicitly in his *Myth of Sisyphus* (*Le mythe de Sisyphe*, 1942), but also in *The Rebel* (*L'homme révolté*, 1951), which attempts to provide a more positive theorization of how to live and act in this state of radical refusal. Plague heightens and dramatizes the fatal predicament in which human life is inextricably bound and trapped. Plague thereby foregrounds and pitilessly reveals some inescapable facts about our mortal, disease-prone condition. Camus suggests that the plague can be revealed as dwelling in us ("chacun la porte en soi, la peste," *La peste*, 228) and as pertaining to our very nature as mortals. Yet it strikes unpredictably and inexorably like a chastisement from heaven overpowering all human efforts to resist or contain it.

Of course, "enlightened" responses resolutely refuse the theologizing that makes humans perversely helpless. Admittedly, brandishing divine punishment as cause has all too often been used as a pretext for neglecting necessary prophylactic measures. However, considering the Enlightenment dialectically, we can hardly refuse to acknowledge that there is also something sound about theological responses in the sense especially of negative theology in recognizing the limits of our human faculties and our being beholden to and dependent on powers beyond our control: *Thanatos*, or death, for one, and *Gaia*, or the earth, for another. Hope, for me, is not to be placed in new vaccines or more sophisticated technologies to render us invulnerable to pandemics but more fundamentally in learning to accept and assume actively and resiliently our constitutive human vulnerability. This is akin to the kind of lesson that I think we might be able to learn from at least some sorts of indigenous cultures, although authority to interpret those traditions I leave with the Indigenous themselves.

3 Myth, History, Fiction, and the Limits of Representation

A negative theology always necessarily entwines itself dialectically with an affirmative theology. Without some "cataphatic" (affirmative) doctrine or description—a concept or image of God—"apophatic" (negative) theology has nothing to negate and cannot be expressed or even register at all. Analogously, the unconditioned absolute that we confront in death and plague issues necessarily in narratives reflecting its impress on our always only relative and partial experience. Obsession with detailed inventory, statistics, bills of mortality, and minute description of symptoms can read as a way of avoiding direct contemplation of the overwhelming facts of massive death and seemingly senseless destruction. Such mayhem, unfiltered, is practically unthinkable. Chronicles and histories are produced, but the litany of facts is never the whole story. History itself becomes an essential medium of revelation of the enigma of life—and death. It is such, notably, in biblical religion, which distinguishes itself from nature religions of neighboring peoples as an *historical* revelation.

Fiction, too, can be a particularly revealing mode of indirect, affirmative expression correlated with the negative theology of the unconditioned, or of the irruption of the unspeakably Other. To call any discourse a "negative theology" simply means that its object or intent—like God—is imagined as infinitely surpassing discourse's own powers of expression. Kafka's fictions—*The Trial, The Castle, The Metamorphosis*, to name only the most familiar—are transparent and programmatic instances of such negative theological imaginings of our being delivered over to irresistible, opaque powers that dominate us all the more implacably the more we struggle against them. Our own will to power is reflected back to us in the inscrutably dominating and menacing specters of the Castle, the Trial, and even the Cockroach.[1]

---

1 I spell this out in the chapter on Kafka in *On What Cannot Be Said: Apophatic Discourses in Philosophy, Religion, Literature, and the Arts*, Edited with Theoretical and Critical Essays by William Franke (Notre Dame: University of Notre Dame Press, 2007), vol. 2, 113–120.

Myth and Fiction work in tandem with History to become channels for raising consciousness of something that remains unrepresentable. It can be apprehended and imagined only through existential or theological lenses refracting how it feels in lived experience. Boccaccio begins from the historical fact of the 1348 plague in Florence as the frame for the one hundred fictions or novellas comprising his *Decameron*. However, in the fictions themselves there is no direct reference to this contextual fact. As historiographer, Boccaccio may well have found himself smack in the middle of this harrowing experience, as certainly his father and family did.[2] He seems to have used fiction as a shield to keep from going mad. He aims to escape through the narrative machine of the ten days and ten novellas per day that nowhere internally allude to the plague. Plague, nevertheless, occasions the whole work and is drawn out graphically in the frame story that relates an actual historical event. This real situation of the historical 1348 Black Death is left deliberately behind by the brigade of seven young women and three young men who leave the city for the surrounding countryside, seeking evasion and relief from omnipresent suffering.

An historical reality is likewise dissimulated, and yet revealed, by fiction in Defoe's *A Journal of the Plague Year*. Although just born in London at the time of the 1665 plague epidemic, Daniel Defoe (1660–1731) writes as a mature first-person, eye-witness narrator, the owner of a saddlery shop, who decides after much hesitation and ambivalence to remain in the city. Incited more directly by the 1720 plague in Marseille, Defoe, as he writes in 1722, is looking back and re-imagining the London plague. He projects himself as a fictive persona into a direct first-person experience of a historical plague by offering searing anecdotes, as well as by meticulously tabulating and comparing the historical records of mortality rates in St Giles and in other heavily stricken parishes.

Alessandro Manzoni, like Defoe, is writing a historical novel at a later time than the event recounted. He takes the historical Milanese plague of 1630 as his material. He works with it in both a historiographical and a fictive mode. He even fuses the two together in the earlier 1827 version of his novel before separating them out later into distinct works, one novelistic (*I promessi sposi*, 1842), the other historiographical (*Storia della Colonna infame*) published as an appendix to the 1842 novel. Both authors employ history and fiction together to create something that is not unequivocally either and that reaches beyond both fact and fantasy to an absolute order of reality. This reality beyond our normal empirical range belongs to a realm accessed rather by religious belief: God is constantly

---

2 The extent to which Boccaccio may have been personally present in Florence during the plague remains a matter of some speculation. See Wayne A. Rebhorn's introduction to the Norton Critical Edition of the *Decameron*, xviii.

evoked both by Defoe's narrator and by Manzoni's characters. Such evocation has a metaphysical air about it.

Without exactly declaring this other reality to be metaphysical, Samuel Weber nevertheless points to the "uncanny" dimension discerned between history and fiction by virtue of their "friction," their rubbing up against and working with, but also against, each other, in plague narratives:

> I will try to characterize these narratives neither as fictional, in the sense of purely imaginary or invented, nor as accurate histories, but as *frictional*. Frictional narratives are both historical and fictional, repetitive and made-up. But this made-up fictional aspect is never absolute, for it involves the way in which the present resonates with the past in anticipating the future. It is this strange mixture of revelation, resonance, and anticipation that tends to comprise every plague, including the coronavirus, which was initially described as being totally "novel" but in the meanwhile seems to have become uncannily familiar. It is this uncanny novelty that calls for a *recounting*.[3]

The noncoinciding relation between the fictional world of the *Decameron* and the surrounding real world in which or out of which it is written is jacked up to an extreme in the tension between the tragically historic plague in Florence and Boccaccio's entertaining stories. Their revelatory power derives to a considerable extent from this discrepancy. Somewhat ambiguously, Boccaccio recalls, in the book's general conclusion, the discrepancy between the work of which he is the author, or rather only the scribe, and God's perfect work of creation:

> But even if one wished to suppose that I was the inventor and the author, which I was not, of those things, I say that I would not be ashamed that all were not pretty since no master can be found, besides God, who does everything well and completely ....
>
> Ma se pur prosuppor si volesse che io fossi stato di quelle e lo 'nventore e lo scrittore, che non fui, dico che io non mi vergognerei che tutte belle non fossero, per ciò che maestro alcun non si truova, da Dio in fuori, che ogni cosa faccia bene e compiutamente ....[4]

Something far beyond Boccaccio's own fictive creation is revealed through its context as framed within the real and historical world that only God can create.

In Boccaccio's medieval worldview, ultimate reality is theological and absolute, and all human reality is but relative. Some such ontological

---

3 Samuel Weber, *Preexisting Conditions: Recounting the Plague*, 25–26.
4 Giovanni Boccaccio, *Il Decamerone*, ed. Vittorio Branca (Milan: Mondadori, 1985), 1111.

difference remains as a residue, I submit, in our discourses concerning plague still in the modern era, even without the metaphysical scaffolding and despite the virtual absorption into one another of history and fiction. Plague remains an indicator of something for which all our modes of discourse are inadequate.

Weber observes that the friction between the real and the fictive is mutually transforming. The stories do not liberate from confinement by the plague, but they do transform it—certainly in the experience of the brigade of youths. The confinement of the ten storytellers in the *Decameron*, Weber observes, takes up elements of an intractable reality in order to "transpose them into a realm where their significance can be altered and developed without being crushed by the weight of reality" (90).

The unbearable burden of the plague is allowed by the indirection of fiction to be expressed by subjects who otherwise could not stand to face it. When Defoe's narrator reports on a nightmarish scene of bodies being carted away and indecorously "shot into the pit, promiscuously" (61) at night amid the indescribable grief of a father and husband for his wife and children, the reality is too much for him to bear and defies representation in the telling: "I was, indeed, shocked with this sight; it almost overwhelmed me; and I went away with my heart most afflicted, and full of afflicting thoughts, such as I cannot describe" (63). The narrator is torn between his irrepressible "curiosity" and his repulsion from such revolting, unendurable scenes. Weber points to the obsession with statistical numbering of the dead and its standing in contradiction with the unique life story behind each death. He teasingly crystalizes this form of unsayability in the paradox of "a story that cannot be tallied, and a tally that cannot be told" (119).

The histories of the plague in London in 1665 and in Milan in 1630 are the basis for the recountings of Defoe and Manzoni respectively. Both straddle historical reporting and the fictionalizing of historical events. History and fiction in modern, highly self-reflective narratives become more and more evidently and consciously inextricable from one another. Both together are used to allude to the unrepresentable—the unfathomable that plague rudely imposes. Myth and Fiction work in tandem with History to become channels for raising consciousness of something that is in itself unrepresentable but pervasively powerful over us. Boccaccio, too, by setting his sometimes frivolous fictions up in counterpoint to the harrowing history of the plague, triangulates History and Fiction on the unrepresentable Other as source of trouble or destruction—but also of hope. Indeed, recreation and renewal have their secret source in the desperate situation in Florence that is abandoned by the brigade retreating to the countryside and to storytelling.

Still, the gnawing question that irrepressibly arises in the face of plague is "Why?" And the hypothesis or disturbing presentiment that plague is caused by higher powers always presses forward in spite of all rationalizing explanations and all reasonable resistance. Exposing humanity as abjectly dependent on and helplessly beholden to some mysterious Power beyond itself is always an upsetting revelation, one unacceptable to most any consistent rationalism. History and fiction working together manage to open within existential reality a space for encounter with something absolute and not accessible within the order either of fact or of fantasy alone. Plague raises the specter of the metaphysical or theological dimension of being or nothingness—to be or not to be—whether interpreted naturalistically or supernaturally.

This is where the symbolic potency of pandemics shows itself as crucial for highlighting their apocalyptic valence as signifying an end to the world as it has been known hitherto. Pandemics necessitate a total reconceptualizing of everything in the world. The myth of Original Sin once again offers an exemplary pattern for the symbolization of pandemics. The world is fallen because of Man's sin spreading as a moral disease infecting all his descendants. The catastrophe is narrativized as an archetypal event, and this changes everything concerning our hopes and expectations for life in this world. The history of apocalyptic in Catholicism and Protestantism, respectively, dramatically illustrates the contrasting potentials of apocalyptic as a narrative paradigm: it can stand for total condemnation and obliteration or for a summons to engagement in and rectification of human history.[5]

---

5 I defer here to my article "Poetics and Apocalypse in Manzoni's Interpretation of History," *Esperienze letterarie* XVIII - n. 4 (1993): 17–38.

4 The Mystery of the Supernatural at the Limit of Naturalism

The dialectic of natural versus supernatural explanations for plagues, which indelibly marks modern treatments, is already discernible in the ancient narratives. It becomes patent when we consider the latter as a dialectical whole. Homer unquestionably attributes the plague to Apollo's arrows. The god is motivated to punish the offense to his divine dignity committed by Agamemnon because the Greek general refuses to honor the suit of Apollo's priest Chryses when the latter brings lavish gifts for the ransom of his daughter Chryseis. Thucydides, in contrast, does not venture to speculate about causes; he leaves that expressly to others (II.48.3). Nonetheless, Thucydides sees pestilence as pushing humanity to its limits and forcing humans to interrogate their why and wherefor. For Sophocles, the plague is visited on Thebes because of Oedipus's transgressions, as revealed by Tiresias the prophet. Seneca's version of this story plays up the supernatural and apocalyptic overtones already clearly sounded in Sophocles. The theological and cosmological contexts are integral to both dramatists' understanding of the cause of pandemic and therefore also of the means for ending it, which consist in correction and in atonement for human transgression. Offenses against the gods and against the moral law, as revealed by Tiresias the prophet, call to be castigated.

Lucretius rejects such theologizing and argues for a purely natural point of view by explaining the plague rationally through his atomic theory ("ratio quae sit morbis … expediam," VI.1090-93). A maleficent combination of atoms or germs causes a contagious miasma that circulates in the air ("semina … quae sint morbo mortique necesse est / multa volare," VI.1093-97). He arrives, nevertheless, at piercing reflections of a metaphysical stamp and tragic in tenor. His poem finishes with a wrenching account of the 430–26 BCE plague that ravaged Athens at the outset of the Peloponnesian War. Dark and sinister overtones threaten to subdue the cheerful, rational serenity that his poem up to this point has promoted. The fact that this devastating description of plague comes at the very end of his epic places his whole optimistic Epicurean philosophy in a much more complex and dubious light than would otherwise be the case. The

DOI: 10.4324/9781003545835-5

plague seems implicitly, by its positioning as the epic's final word, to call into question the efficacy of the Epicurean ethics of disciplined self-control for maximizing pleasure and well-being that have been extolled throughout the work. The discourse of the poem is overwhelmed and reduced to silence by the plague at its end: we contemplate a nothingness beyond the intricate—but in this light artificial—system of thought that Lucretius has constructed.

A divergence of interpretations—naturalistic versus supernatural, purely human versus mythical and theological—opens up between Lucretius and his heirs, Virgil and Ovid. The latter, while working closely with the Lucretian model, reverse its scientific naturalism. They insert their descriptions into elaborate mythological contexts, evoking the agency of the gods and their superhuman motivations and machinations.

This tension is accentuated in modern secular culture and becomes more conscious and explicit, often demanding an agonizing choice between points of view. The ancient authors seem not to be so perplexed by alternative, contradictory outlooks. Still, regardless of whether it elicits a metaphysical or merely a medical regard, plague is apt to occasion a more searching self-examination and exposure of the paradoxes and contradictions of human life. Already Thucydides, in his relatively dispassionate account (by comparison with his Latin imitators), extends an explicit invitation to see clearly in past events what human nature itself prepares for the future (I, 22). Plague strips away the veneer from what civilization conceals, exposing its subterfuges, and reveals human nature nakedly to itself.

Likewise, the *Decameron*'s more emotionally involved, grave, and pathetic account of the plague emphasizes, above all, how it forces us to face up to some unseemly truths about our humanity that society in its normal functioning is well organized to mask and dissemble. All sense of decency is lost and the dignity of persons is completely violated as cadavers are heaped up together in piles. Basic bonds of kinship and community cease to function in face of the terror of the Black Death. Corpses are dumped into ditches without customary funeral rites. When normal social order breaks down, a savageness in us is unconcealed. Certain truths are revealed about life and death—but also about the social and imaginative constructions that are ingeniously or deviously designed to hide and disguise appalling propensities of an only superficially civilized humanity.

The *Decameron*'s first novella is about a rogue, Ser Ciappelletto, whose death and glorification illustrate how a saint can be manufactured through the social construction of public knowledge made, in good part, out of mendaciously fabricated information and also, in part, from innocent credulity. The grotesque deception, nonetheless, redounds to God's greater glory. The Almighty can use even such corrupt means for the purpose of engendering pious faith and a spirit of sacrifice in those who are made devout and who make virtuous vows thanks even to Ciappelletto's most thoroughly vicious, however apparently holy, exemplar. Boccaccio even allows in the end that, hidden in God's judgment, Ciappelletto may really be a saint after all, based on some genuine last-minute act of contrition!

This concluding remark, of course, is bitingly ironic, and yet it does accurately acknowledge and pivot on the difference between all finite, human understanding and the infinite understanding that would be God's. By means of this relation, Boccaccio effectively places his writing in the purview of an infinite divine Mind that contrasts with his own finite mind and fleeting existence. He has invoked this all-encompassing will and superior intelligence in contrast to worldly transience already in the Prologue (*Proemio*): "But just as it pleased Him who, being himself infinite, gave as an immutable law to all worldly things to have an end ..." ("Ma sì come a Colui piacque il quale, essendo Egli infinito, diede per legge incommutabile a tutte le cose mondane aver fine ...").[1] Again, the ontological and metaphysical difference between human experience and divine mystery is made palpable by the limit-experience of plague.

God's governance of the universe is without appeal and beyond question. And so, the "just anger of God" ("giusta ira di Dio") is evoked as the plague's Cause from the first day and its "horrid beginning" ("orrido comminciamento"). Nonetheless, Boccaccio seems to leave open the possibility also of a natural cause: "whether through malignant influence of the stars or as just punishment for human iniquity" ("o per operazion de' corpi superiori o per le nostre inique opere").[2] However, the stars, too, are superhuman and generally thought to be divinely guided, and Boccaccio quickly returns to his wrath-of-God hypothesis ("l'ira di Dio") without expressing any uncertainty but only scorn for those who thought they could escape the plague by leaving the city, as if its walls could circumscribe the reach of divine retribution.

Defoe's narrator is similarly convinced that the plague is a punishment from God, but many of his interlocutors do not share this conviction. The narrator admits that even "My brother, though a very religious man himself, laughed at all I had suggested about its being an intimation from Heaven, and told me several stories of such foolhardy people ... as I was; ...."[3]

---

1 Boccaccio, *Decamerone*, 7.
2 Boccaccio, *Decamerone*, 12, 16.
3 Daniel Defoe, *Journal of the Plague Year*, first published March 17, 1722, available online at Internet Archive and Gutenberg as: "A Journal of the Plague Year, Being Observations or Memorials, Of the most Remarkable Occurrences, As well Publick as Private, which happened in *London*, During the last Great Visitation in 1665, Written by a Citizen who continued all the while in London. Never made public before," ed. George Rice Carpenter (New York: Longmans, Green, and Co., 1896), 14. Accessed from www.gutenberg.com on 3/6/2023.

Those who opt for a purely naturalistic explanation and understanding of events confidently deride the narrator for his religious convictions concerning the plague. They vent their scorn even to the point of blasphemy:

> But that which was the worst in all their devilish language was, that they were not afraid to blaspheme God and talk atheistically, making a jest of my calling the plague the hand of God; mocking, and even laughing, at the word judgement, as if the providence of God had no concern in the inflicting such a desolating stroke; and that the people calling upon God as they saw the carts carrying away the dead bodies was all enthusiastic, absurd, and impertinent.[4]

The Defoean narrator's religious faith is severely put to the test by the Black Death and its unrelenting horror. Still, he resolves, rather than flee, to stay in the city and to commend himself with trust entirely into the hands of God, for, as the Psalmist says,

> Surely he shall deliver thee from the snare of the fowler, and from the noisome pestilence.... Thou shalt not be afraid for the terror by night; nor for the arrow that flieth by day; nor for the pestilence that walketh in darkness; nor for the destruction that wasteth at noonday. A thousand shall fall at thy side, and ten thousand at thy right hand; but it shall not come nigh thee ... there shall no evil befall thee; neither shall any plague come nigh thy dwelling.[5]

This personal faith of the narrator's contrasts with the more rational and skeptical mindset of those around him. He trusts, instead, in his piety to protect him against the worst ravages of the plague. Whatever the narrator's opinions and those of his critics may be, whether theistic or naturalistic, superstitious or rationalist, the plague theme appeals to a kind of apocalyptic imagination of the world coming to its end. No matter how one chooses to explain and deal with it, plague prompts imaginings of extreme conditions that place us face to face with the limits of life and of common humanity.

In his age of greater social consensus and collective consciousness, Boccaccio could assume that the plague would be intelligibly interpreted

---

4 Defoe, *Journal*, 66.
5 Defoe, *Journal*, 16. Psalms 91:3-7, King James Version. It should be noted that Luther had made *not* fleeing from plague into a Christian's duty if staying would serve one's community. Martin Luther, "Ob man vor dem Sterben fliehen möge" (1552), in *Ausgewählte Schriften*, vol. 2, ed. Hans Christian Knuth (Frankfurt am Main: Insel Verlag, 2016), trans. Carl J. Schindler, "Whether One May Flee From a Deadly Plague" (1527), in *Luther's Works*, vol. 43, *Devotional Writings*, ed. Gustav K. Wiencke (Philadelphia: Fortress Press, 1968).

as a punishment from God for the sins of the city of Florence made haughty by its newfound wealth and power. Its unprecedented success seduces the unwary city into moral laxity and turpitude that render it deserving of divine chastisement. But in Defoe's Enlightenment-era London such an interpretation could not but be highly contested. A rationalist view refusing unscientific explanations scornfully confronts such a traditional religious understanding.

5 From Ambiguity of Causes to Moral Certitude through Existential Conversion

Manzoni's treatment swings ambiguously between consistent rationalism and a more mystic-apocalyptic vision of the historical significance of the plague. Paradoxically, driven by fear, rationalism itself can become irrational and fanatical. The preference of the larger, seventeenth-century public as represented in the novel—but surely also as reflecting Manzoni's own nineteenth-century audience—is for attributing the plague to tangible causes that can be combatted, specifically the "smearers" (*untori*) or poisoners:

> The minds of the people, ever more embittered by the presence of the evil, irritated by the insistence of the danger, embraced the more willingly that belief: for anger aims to punish: and ... prefers to attribute the evils to human perversity, against which it is possible to take revenge, rather than to recognize them as coming from a cause to which one can do nothing other than resign oneself.
>
> Gli animi, sempre più amareggiati dalla presenza de' mali, irritati dall'insistenza del pericolo, abbracciavano più volentieri quella credenza: ché la collera aspira a punire: e ... le piace più d'attribuire i mali a una perversità umana, contro cui possa far le sue vendette, che di riconoscerli da una causa, con la quale non ci sia altro da fare che rassegnarsi.[1]

On the other hand, putative religious causes of plague, when treated too positively, also stand under accusation. Manzoni deplores the public penance drawn out in a religious procession with the relics of Saint Carlo Borromeo (1538–84). The saint was widely revered for combatting a previous bout of plague in Milan, to which he nonetheless fell victim. This public spectacle was demanded by popular sentiment as a measure to placate divine anger and, hopefully, allay the plague. It was allowed

---

1 Manzoni, *I promessi sposi* (Milan: Mondadori, 1985), 714–715.

only against the better judgment of the ecclesiastic in office, Federigo Borromeo, the great saint's spiritual successor and heir. This surge of demonstrative, public piety is shown to be a sort of irrational, emotional behavior designed to concretize the evil in some tangible form, even if it is only a symbolic ritual. This type of reification is all-too-endemic to the minds—and especially the emotions—of popular masses. The result, predictably, is exponential aggravation of the contagion.

Manzoni (1785–1873) is himself, at times, an integrally Enlightenment thinker—but at other times he is incorrigibly Romantic. He was educated in eighteenth-century Enlightenment ideals but was soon swept up in the Romantic currents of his age. He laments the tragedy that is caused by such superstitious, popular belief with its heavy toll of deaths. He caustically exposes the absurd folly of astrological approaches to accounting for the plague. His satire on the figure of Don Ferrante, culminating in the penultimate chapter (XXXVII) of the novel, discharges this latter function with superbly sardonic wit.

Manzoni faults the public authorities for not minding the medical experts who issued warnings about the plague. He derisively details the slow and painful process of gradually, reluctantly coming to recognition and avowal that indeed it was *plague* and not something else less frightening. For far too long the official discourse maintained that it was "not truly plague, that is to say, plague, yes, but in a certain manner of speaking; not plague proper, but something for which we are not able to find another name" ("Poi, non vera peste, vale a dire peste sì, ma in un certo senso; non peste proprio, ma una cosa alla quale non si sa trovare un altro nome"). Precious time was squandered before the final admission that indeed *plague* was wreaking havoc, causing death and disruption of people's lives throughout the region of Milan.[2] The idea that human expertise and effective action can master such menaces reflects Manzoni's faith in reason and a conviction that we must manage such problems.

Yet those who do manage to positively confront the pandemic—exemplarily brother Cristoforo—are religious, saintly figures resigned to die in self-sacrifice for the salvation of others. They conquer themselves and thereby convert the hearts of others, even while succumbing physically to the irresistible virulence of the pandemic. The vision of history underlying the entire novel is ultimately a Christian providential vision, and this in the end colors its presentation of the plague. This Christian providential perspective is fideistic, based on an "indeterminate faith" ("fiducia indeterminata," 477) rather than on any demonstrable certitudes (Illustration 5.1).

---

2 Manzoni, *I promessi sposi*, Chapter XXXI, 449.

32 *Pandemics and Apocalypse in World Literature*

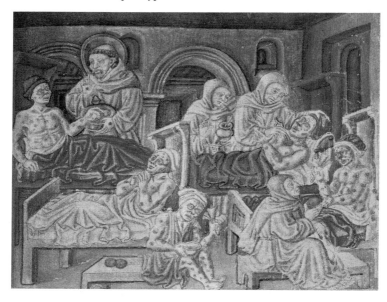

Illustration 5.1 "Franciscan monks treating victims of the plague," Jacopo Oddi (d. 1474).

For all his meticulous tracing of causes, Manzoni also recognizes the ostensibly arbitrary nature of the contagion that comes and goes like the rain (chapter XXXVII) in spite of all that humans can do. This acknowledgment of the incalculable and inscrutable, which the pandemic makes us face, together with the uselessness of all human measures against it, comes back, and presses forward, in all our authors, religious or not. Thucydides, Lucretius, and Ovid all emphasize the utter cluelessness of medical science to comprehend and combat the plague:

> Neither could the physicians do anything; they did not know this disease and found themselves treating it for the first time. Instead, they themselves died most rapidly since they most neared the sick, nor could any other human art do any better. Any prayers of supplication in temples or proclaiming of divinations proved equally futile. The overwhelming disaster put an end to all such attempts.
>
> οὔτε γὰρ ἰατροὶ ἤρκουν τὸ πρῶτον θεραπεύοντες ἀγνοίᾳ, ἀλλ' αὐτοὶ μάλιστα ἔθνῃσκον ὅσῳ καὶ μάλιστα προσῇσαν, οὔτε ἄλλη ἀνθρωπεία

τέχνη οὐδεμία: ὅσα τε πρὸς ἱεροῖς ἱκέτευσαν ἢ μαντείοις καὶ τοῖς τοιούτοις ἐχρήσαντο, πάντα ἀνωφελῆ ἦν, τελευτῶντές τε αὐτῶν ἀπέστησαν ὑπὸ τοῦ κακοῦ νικώμενοι.
–Thucydides, *History of the Peloponnesian War* II.47.4

Lucretius, too, admits that the physicians are dumbfounded and immobilized by their consternation faced with the disease:

"Medicine stood paralyzed in silent fear."

("Mussabat tacito medicina timore")
Lucretius, *De rerum natura*, VI.1179

No rational remedy for the disease can be found ("Nec ratio remedi communis certa dabatur," *De rerum natura*, VI.1226).

Ovid suggests that attempts to combat the plague were based on ignorance of its supernatural cause, namely, the anger of the goddess Juno on account of Jupiter's infidelities:

As long as the disaster seemed of human origin and the cause
of so much death remained hidden, medical art was deployed against it;
but the scourge exceeded the ability to resist, which lay vanquished.

Dum visum mortale malum tantaeque latebat
Causa nocens cladis, pugnatum est arte medendi;
Exitium superabat opem, quae victa iacebat.
– Ovid, *Metamorphoses*, VII.525-27

Even Virgil, always highly metaphorical and mythological, very little adherent to plain fact, notes that all human arts only made things worse ("quasitaeque nocent artes") and that the master physicians simply gave up ("cessere magistri," *Georgics* III.549).

Boccaccio, too, repeats this trope of the utter incapacity and unpreparedness of physicians and their medical arts to cope with this health crisis coming from the Orient and essentially unknown in its causes ("A cura delle quali infermità né consiglio di medico né virtù di medicina alcuna pareva che valesse o facesse profitto ... non conoscesse da che si movesse," 13). This is what Walter Benjamin calls being without a clue, "Ratlosigkeit," literally, "without counsel."[3] The plague and its epic-novelistic, as well as its journalistic, narration consistently leads to this impasse.

I underscore this impasse as forcing a certain opening to a realm of the absolute—what religious faith or poetic vision has always perceived as a

---

3 See Weber, *Preexisting Conditions*, 31, on Benjamin's theory of the Story-Teller or *Erzähler*.

source of inspiration transcending human powers. Weber, following Benjamin, apprehends this dimension as "uncanny." This sets up the situation of narrative openness that Benjamin theorizes as characteristic of "storytelling," which always invites new departures and never comes to a final conclusion, as do epics and novels. Weber's relating plague to "storytelling" gives its processing this dimension of formal openness that, I have stressed, is engendered more deeply and concretely and existentially by human helplessness vis-à-vis an absoluteness about the real.

This ancient theme of human helplessness as revealed by plague is common to all our accounts regardless of whether their authors are religiously inclined or strictly secular. The surpassing of human capacities opens a dimension of the "beyond" that is bound to be inhabited and invested by hope and/or despair. The same mystery as surrounds the cause and origins in the ancient and medieval texts continues to envelop especially the accounts of the relenting and cessation of pandemics in modern texts. Remission of the pestilence lies beyond human control and is experienced as a kind of miracle of grace.

Defoe's narrator is thankful to God "our Preserver" for finally putting a stop to the "dreadful calamity." He is convinced that

> Nothing but the immediate finger of God, nothing but omnipotent power, could have done it. The contagion despised all medicine; death raged in every corner; and had it gone on as it did then, a few weeks more would have cleared the town of all, and everything that had a soul.... In that very moment when we might very well say, 'Vain was the help of man',—I say, in that very moment it pleased God, with a most agreeable surprise, to cause the fury of it to abate, even of itself.
>
> (*Journal of the Plague Year*, 249)

The unaccountability of the plague's relenting is for this narrator incontrovertible proof of the supernatural hand of God at work:

> The disease was enervated and its malignity spent; and let it proceed from whencesoever it will, let the philosophers search for reasons in nature to account for it by, and labour as much as they will to lessen the debt they owe to their Maker, those physicians who had the least share of religion in them were obliged to acknowledge that it was all supernatural, that it was extraordinary, and that no account could be given of it.
>
> (*Journal of the Plague Year*, 251)

Even from his position poles apart from the Defoe narrator's piety, Camus makes the same observation that the plague departed as unaccountably as it had arrived. The human measures that had previously been impotent to prevent its fatal spread suddenly became effective as the plague lost its momentum (245). In the end, in every historical instance described in our literary specimens, plague simply peters out, slacking of its own accord. It is not mastered. Instead, one day, when this result is least expected, the pandemic has simply expended itself. It ends not with a bang but a whimper.

6 Securing Control versus Acknowledging Grace and Vulnerability

The irony of such unaccountable outcomes to plague epidemics is intuited and deployed fictively by H. G. Wells in *The War of the Worlds* (1897). Wells's Martians, after overcoming human resistance by force of arms and conquering the earth, fall victim to disease caused by pathogenic microbes to which they have no immunity. The invaders from outer space are "slain by the putrefactive and disease bacteria against which their systems were unprepared; … slain, after all man's devices had failed, by the humblest things that God, in his wisdom, has put upon this earth."[1] So the Martian threat, like the plague, simply disappears after all human efforts to resist it have proved futile. Plague or pandemic exceeds the control even of superhuman Martians, who were able to subdue all human force: it comes and goes uncontrollably, regardless of anyone's bidding.

Rather than fight it, Boccaccio's approach is to exit the impossible situation posed by a hostile nature and enter into the pure artifice of telling stories. The mysteries of providence and punishment cannot be mastered humanly. All that Boccaccio and his characters can do is look away and entertain themselves while hoping that it will pass. There is surely some wisdom in this approach, too. It entails keeping our spirits up as best we can, through art and games and the artificial ordering of our lives, while making room for a destiny that we do not fully control to play itself out. This is the wisdom that Kafka's anxious protagonist K is lacking. It is our pretense to total control of our destiny that itself gives its energy to the plague also in a work such as Camus's *La peste*, where the public health catastrophe, combined with the countermeasures designed to contain it, serves as an allegory for a fascist regime. This approach, of course, is liable to be suspected of being fatalistic. It treats plague as a divine or irrational mystery rather than as a human responsibility.

---

1 H. G. Wells, *The War of the Worlds* (London: Chapman and Hall, 1897), Book 2 (The Earth Under the Martians), Chapter 8 (Dead London), 5. Žižek, *Pandemic: COVID-19 Shakes the World*, 12–13, mentions this suggestive instance from popular science fiction.

DOI: 10.4324/9781003545835-7

Roland Barthes sharply criticized Camus for dehistoricizing and even dehumanizing the plague under the figure of a goddess acting like an ancient Fate who is unknowable ("One knows nothing of her except that she *is*").[2] The very genre of myth, or at least Camus's use of it, is censured as mystification. Jean-Paul Sartre and Simone de Beauvoir expressed similar dissatisfaction and indignation, lending these criticisms a more aggressively polemical edge. With sufficient historical distance, however, current criticism reverses this judgment and finds precisely here the novel's crucial function of phenomenological revealment.

At stake in Camus's plague is the unrepresentable or even the unspeakable of the Shoah (colloquially known as the "brown plague"): evoking this unsayability is the author's task, even before furnishing human directives for coping with specific political issues. Anjuli Fatima Raza Kolb suggests that

> What might have been depicted as a frontal event in which the healthy city faces the enemy of plague, like so many soldiers approaching from just beyond the horizon, is instead represented as an emergent event that can be known only through its effects and may not yet be nameable, may even, as we have seen, be unthinkable.[3]

Camus opens access to a metaphysical, or at least not fully manifest, aspect of this unthinkable "event" as only "emergent."

Camus struck a nerve with this book in its 1947 context, one that became live with us again after the unlimited vulnerability discovered through the September 11, 2001, terrorist attacks on the World Trade Center and the Pentagon.[4] Is it the West's attempt to control the world that itself provokes such unpreventable attacks against it? The effort to control ineluctably engenders resistance. Transposed imaginatively into literature, this, again, is the type of question that doggedly pursues K in Kafka's novels. The more any rational reduction of the causes is applied, so that the evil agents can supposedly be crushed or expunged, the less it works and the more this effort brings about effects opposite to its aims. What is called for, instead, is an openness of spirit for meeting with and attempting to understand the Other, which—or who—is ultimately to be acknowledged as an unsoundable mystery demanding unconditional respect.

---

2 Roland Barthes, "La *Peste*: Annales d'une épidémique ou roman de solitude?" *Club*, February 1955: 6, *Œuvres complètes*, 540–541.

3 Anjuli Fatima Raza Kolb, *Epidemic Empire: Colonialism, Contagion, and Terror, 1817-2020* (Chicago: University of Chicago Press, 2021), 129–169, chapter 4: The Brown Plague. Citation 150.

4 Tony Judt, "On 'The Plague,'" *New York Review of Books* (November 29, 2001), gives a good sense of this shifting context. http://www.nyb00ks.com/articles/archives/2001/n0v/29/0n-the-plague/.

The overarching issue raised for human communities and commonwealths by plague, according to these narratives across the centuries, is whether plague is to be attributed to inscrutable causes in heaven or whether human beings should be held responsible for producing it—or at least for finding out its causes and taking the appropriate preventative and curative, and perhaps even punitive, measures. However, this simple opposition between an obscurantist religious and a scientifically enlightened approach breaks down with thoroughgoing examination and reflection on the literature. Somehow, rational response needs to be articulated alongside and be coordinated with acknowledgment of its limits.

What plague or pandemic, together with the human reaction to it, discloses is a dimension in which our existence is grounded above itself and beyond our control. We are made to face our radical non-sovereignty over ourselves and our lives and our vulnerability to disease and ultimately death. Admission of this condition of our existence is perennially difficult for us to accept and deal with. This contingent predicament of our life never fails to perplex us. We can deny it, or we can fanatically fixate on it. In either case, like Kafka's K, we make it worse, compounding its complexity and our own perplexity, and we are often spurred to act in drastic and even desperate ways, upsetting nature's equilibrium and our own.

By my emphasis on our non-sovereignty, I do not mean to suggest that we cannot and should not strive to be sovereign over certain spheres and aspects of our existence. But the whole of our existence and its ultimate end exceeds our control: we are obliged to open up to something or someone Other if we want to relate as whole beings to the real as a whole. This is the existential posture that modern techno-scientific culture is generally geared to refusing and denying. Covid-19, like plagues throughout history, functions as a reminder of this preexisting condition, this *conditionedness*, from which we otherwise strive in every way to escape.

Like Manzoni, Camus emphasizes the slowness and reluctance of the authorities to face the facts and acknowledge that what they are up against is indeed the "plague," calling it by its true name (*La peste*, 49–52). It is simply too terrifying to find oneself overtaken and participating directly in the unimaginable horror of the "great plagues of history" ("grandes pestes de l'histoire," 45). In both Manzoni's and Camus's fictions, the public authorities are accused of tardiness and are convicted by the facts of "insufficiency" in the measures taken. However, the real difficulty is that no measures whatever can be even remotely "sufficient" against plague. The cowardly refusal to admit the true nature of the epidemic certainly deserves to be denounced and reprimanded. Yet, reticence can also be motivated by the desire to preserve the public from panic, which helps no one and can swiftly turn into a deadly public health hazard in its own right. The dilemma is that, howsoever lucid it may be, a designation of the problem as "plague" is also tantamount to an admission of helplessness to prevent or even substantially mitigate it. Furthermore, there are always good scientific grounds for incertitude, and hence hesitation, regarding any phenomenon as complex and elusive as plague. In this regard, "plague," as the word comes down to us through its rich literary tradition, connotes primarily the limits of human abilities to cope.

Manzoni, in the Romantic Age, had experienced the limits of Enlightenment rationalism, while Camus, as a twentieth-century existentialist, was in revolt against the limits of scientific positivism and its totalizing rationality. Both authors castigate the lack of prompt and adequate reaction to the initial indicators of plague, exposing typical human hypocrisies and tergiversations. Yet both are far from affirming that resolute rational action is all that is called for to get things under control and save the day. Finding a practical fix or technical remedy for the crisis is not their focus. The conscious awareness that they both inculcate reaches immeasurably further. They open a visionary, apocalyptic purview in which the unsurpassable limits of humanity and its mortality are soberingly contemplated.

Although in many pandemic narratives the supernatural explanations are subjected to serious, even scathing critique, as well as to ironic ridicule, nevertheless the narratives in every instance cannot help but acknowledge and expose something far beyond human control as emerging in and through the catastrophe of the Black Death or other pandemics. We are rudely reminded that, in any case, death and vulnerability to disease designate a limit to our control. It is this confrontation with the absolute negation of human sovereignty, our being forced to face our impotence and death, that is their common denominator. This constitutes essentially an apocalyptic revelation to which the literary renderings of pandemics in one way or another all attest.

Learning to accept and cope with this degree of crisis reaching to the foundations of our existence is a mighty challenge. One does not have to believe in otherworldly instances or the supernatural: it is enough to be confronted with the radical alterity of the other person who exists beyond our control. This unsurpassable limit to our sovereignty poses nearly insuperable difficulties for us to learn to accept. Especially the wars raging in our own time (from the Ukraine and Palestine to Yemen and the Sudan) witness to this basic difficulty of acknowledging and coexisting with others.[5] Affirmation of self, when fixed within a finite horizon eclipsing sight of our common root in the In-finite (or in what no language or culture can adequately define), tragically results in suppression of the Other and of all that is other.

---

5 For further reflection on war in the philosophical perspective being developed here, I defer to my article "Not War, Nor Peace. Are War and Peace Mutually Exclusive Alternatives?" *War: Thinking the Unthinkable*, eds. Cindy Zeiher and Mike Grimshaw, Special Issue of *Continental Thought and Theory: A Journal of Intellectual Freedom* 4/1 (2023): 25–35.

7 Hope in a Negative Theological and Apocalyptic-Fictive Register of Wholeness

While this avowal of impotence may seem to be a note of hopelessness—and is such for our ability to control and dominate pandemics by our technological means—I suggest that this limit of our human powers is precisely where we should search for motives for sustainable hope in a negative theological register. There is a more authentic dimension of our being human than that of managing innerworldly threats and crises. Making precisely a quantum leap into this higher dimension of what we might call "transhumanity" (in the sense of Dante's "trasumanar" in *Paradiso* I.70) is at stake in our confrontation with pandemics as mediated by visionary literary texts. Dante's *trasumanar*, which "cannot be signified verbally" ("trasumanar significar per verba non si poría"), intends a transformative relation to a divine Other. Dante's mystic ascent to the vision of God is practically the opposite of the current transhumanist agenda of rendering humanity absolutely autonomous and immune even to death. This latter type of transhumanism (the common one today) aims to overcome our dependence on anything other than ourselves by our own power and technology and to render the human being invulnerable. This constitutes an idolatry of our particular material organism, perpetuating mere life of individual bodies separated from the continuum of life as a whole.[1]

Already in the current crisis, the imperative embraced by governments of preserving human lives at all costs absolutizes and idolatrizes life in the manifest form of individual bodies and blinds us to a human life's relation to anything greater than itself, for the sake of which it might even be sacrificed. In an exceptionally lucid book on the Covid-19 crisis, not without some strong resonances with the writings of Giorgio Agamben, Olivier Rey pertinently analyzes as "idolatry" our governments' and public health systems' placing supreme importance on the absolute imperative enjoining the preservation of mere life ("la vie nue") abstracted from all its actual

---

1 Olivier Rey, *Leurre et malheur du transhumanisme* (Paris: Desclée de Brouwer, 2018) offers a cogent critique of transhumanism in such terms.

DOI: 10.4324/9781003545835-8

content and qualities and isolated from its intrinsic value.[2] For lack of recognition of any true or transcendent absolute or higher value, life itself in the concrete form of individual bodies is absolutized.[3] This reifying habit of mind gives tangible shape also to the opposite of life—death or disease—as an identifiable and expugnable "enemy." Such positivistic perception has become glaringly dominant in our late modernity with its technological apocalypse. Can ancient wisdom possibly serve us as a corrective?

My orientation to a life beyond the life of the individual body might be considered Lucretian in tenor and be worked out in materialist terms. Judith Butler writes, "Call me a Lucretian," in observing that "The pandemic upends our usual sense of the bounded self, casting us as relational, interactive, and refuting the egological and self-interested bases of ethics itself" (11–12). This is the point on which my reflection turns in appropriating the ancient philosopher's essential vision of "the nature of things" (*rerum natura*). I aim to assimilate something unexpectedly valuable also from the other classic texts that I review: they can be highly instructive about our present predicament because they speak from outside the systematically distorted communications that arise in any large-scale crisis management situation.

Just as public pressure during the plagues described by our classic authors produced presumably guilty parties as scapegoats, so governments today are practically forced to pretend to find the guilty party and take measures to extirpate it.[4] We are "at war" against the virus, as the French president Emanuel Macron declared ("nous sommes en guerre"). And we have weapons in the form of vaccines to kill or, at any rate, disarm it. But, in ways intolerable for many, these means are also apt to kill and mutilate us and our own social, civic, cultural, and economic life. The measures taken serve, perhaps chiefly, to create the appearance that the public authorities are in control of the situation, that they have placed the responsible parties under arrest or declared war against them.

In the introduction to the "History of the Infamous Column," Manzoni avows that all of the errors of the Milanese judges could not be attributed to honest mistakes but were perverted by iniquitous passions ("non si posson riferir ad altro che a passioni pervertitrici della volontà")

---

2 Olivier Rey, *L'idolâtrie de la vie* (Paris: Gallimard, 2020), 31–36.
3 Saitya Brata Das, *Political Theology of Life* (Eugene: Pickwick, 2023) develops such an argument by apophatic lights, resourcing Eckhart, Schelling, and Kierkegaard.
4 René Girard, *Le bouc émissaire* (Paris: Grasset, 1982), chapter 1 on Guillaume de Machaut, *Jugement dou Roy de Navarre*, analyzes the scapegoat mechanism in medieval attributions of the Black Death to the Jews. His theory has been applied specifically to the Covid-19 pandemic by Adriano Vinale, "Epidemiologia politica: Foucault, Girard e la pandemia da Covid-19," *Storia e politica* 12/3 (2020): 416–436.

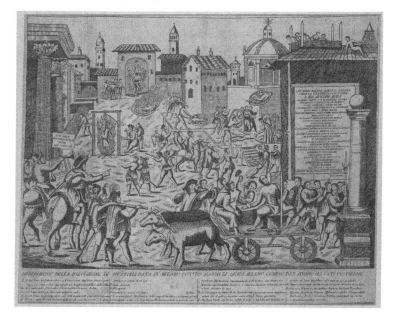

Illustration 7.1 "Torture and execution of 'anointers' in 1630 Milanese plague," Anon.

(Illustration 7.1).[5] Manzoni's anatomy of how the judges were dominated by irrational passions of anger and fear ("quella rabbia e quel timore," *Storia della colonna infame*, 4) is all too revealing of how all-too-human emotions guided the responses to Covid-19. Since the crisis, backlash against Dr. Anthony Fauci (then-Chief Medical Advisor to the President) in the United States and Dr. Karl Lauterbach (Minister of Health) in Germany has been merciless and unsparing.[6] Accusations against the authorities for lying to conserve and exert power refuse to subside. There was also often a tendency to blame the pandemic, or its persistence, on the minorities refusing the vaccine, for whatever reasons—the so-called "no vax" or "anti-vax," who lost their jobs or licenses to practice or rights to frequent public spaces. These defensive and aggressive reactions focused on delivering a scapegoat can blind us to the revelation of the need to

---

5 Alessandro Manzoni, *Storia della colonna infame*, ed. Ferruccio Ulivi (Rome: Newton Compton, 1993), 3–4.
6 Lauterbach Warum Deutschland die Pandemie ohne ihn beendet | Inside PolitiX - YouTube and Attacks on Fauci grow more intense, personal and conspiratorial - POLITICO. Accessed 17-5-2023.

radically amend our lifestyle and to drastically scale back our disastrous impact on the natural environment.

The blindness to our own perverse ways is fostered and protected by a kind of witch-hunt that prevents us from seeing what we can and need to do to rectify the ethical imbalances and disequilibrium in which we are living, or rather dying. Even the necessary and legitimate defensive measures of the public health authorities are apt to be ensconced in metaphorical, fantastic narratives of combatting an enemy. They thereby gain in force and motivation in the manner of populist propaganda.

The sad and even horrendous truth made manifest by Manzoni's careful examination of justice in times of plague is that laws and institutions serve as instruments in the hands of gangs holding power to impose their own prejudices and preferences as right and just. This intricate exposé of certain human perversities triggered by the disaster is continuous with Manzoni's more metaphysical revelation on an altogether higher level of his epic fiction.

Fiction, or symbolic narrative, is an apt vehicle for this higher or deeper, apocalyptic dimension of revelation. Without fiction, there can be no theology. Since God is per se unknowable, whatever we say about God is always a rendering by imaginative means of our relation to something in itself unknowable and yet absolutely conditioning for us—something ineluctable throughout our practical lives.

I turn to what we classify as fiction or imaginative literature in the conviction that, as Victor Hugo observed, legend is not less true than history, nor history less false than legend ("la légende est aussi fausse et aussi vraie que l'histoire").[7] Fiction may be even more revealing than fact of our ultimate possibilities. Aristotle placed poetic truth higher than the truth of history because of its capacity for revealing universal rather than just particular truths (*Poetics* 1451b). But a negative poetics opening to what is beyond its range of representation can fathom the universality that is not (anything definable).[8] By means of poetry, we can relate negatively to this (Un)ground from which truth and everything else comes.

Self-critically aware of itself as fiction, fiction can make room for a truth or reality that exceeds all possibilities that can be imagined and expressed, a kind of "beyond" of truth. As Mark Twain wittily quips: "Truth is stranger than fiction, but it is because Fiction is obliged to stick to possibilities; Truth isn't."[9] In becoming self-critical, fiction can reach out beyond itself, and beyond all conceivable possibilities, to truth. It can

---

7 Victor Hugo, *Quatrevingt-Treize* (1874): projet de préface.
8 For further elucidation, see my *On the Universality of What Is Not: The Apophatic Turn in Critical Thinking* (Notre Dame: University of Notre Dame Press, 2020).
9 Mark Twain, *Following the Equator: A Journey Around the World* (Hartford: American Publishing Company, 1897), 156.

44 *Pandemics and Apocalypse in World Literature*

open a space even for the truth that it cannot represent or imagine. I turn, then, to theology as a sublime and eminently revealing *fictio* that is peculiarly suited for sounding the depths of being and the ultimate conditions of our existence by relating us—in its apophatic form as negative theology—to the real or divine as the unthinkable and whole beyond the range of our wildest imaginings.

Plagues and epidemics have produced a great deal of fictions such as William Maxwell's *They Came Like Swallows* (1938) and Katherine Anne Porter's *Pale Horse, Pale Rider* (1939). Both are about the Spanish flu pandemic in 1918–19 that proved to be a fathomless revelation of human beings to themselves. Self-critically aware of itself as fiction, fiction can make room for a truth or reality that exceeds all possibilities that can be imagined and expressed. It can figure inextinguishable relationships—of the dying mother with her family, for example, in Maxwell's novel. This fiction figures a dimension of infinite openness to one another in emotion which knows no limits (Illustration 7.2).

Reference to the Book of Revelation, which features a pale horse whose rider is death (6:7-8), is frequent in this literature. Apocalypse, as revelation of the alpha and the omega, first and last (Revelation 12:13),

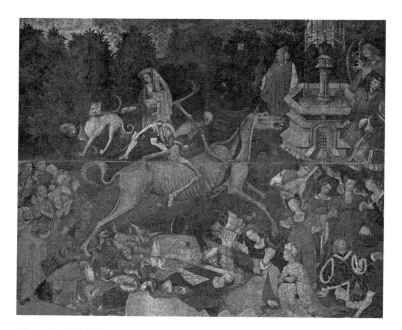

Illustration 7.2 "Triumph of Death," unknown master, Palazzo Abbatellis, Palermo, 1446.

the whole, constitutes a fundamental parameter for reflection on the entire cluster of phenomena relating to plagues and pandemics. The word "apocalypse" connotes both universal destruction, such as pandemics usher in for all (*pan*) people (*demos*), and also a religious revelation or apocalypse of ultimate mysteries concerning "last things," which are brought out (*apo*) of concealment (*calypso*). In either case, the end of the world as we have known it is announced. It is this conjunction between the threat of a generalized, systemic collapse represented by pandemic and the total revelation of the real in apocalypse that is the focus of these reflections on the Covid-19 pandemic in a world-historical and literary perspective as turning on a kind of (non)revelation of humanity to itself. I say "non" because, in an apophatic perspective, what is revealed is a certain unrevealability that induces rather to an openness to the All and the Other more than to disclosing a definite object that would be unveiled.

A salient feature of pandemics is the stripping away of the veil of ordinary life that blinds us to ultimate meanings—as well as to the meaninglessness or annihilation which can serve as their ground. We can discover this at many different levels and in different ways as we move through the representations of pandemic disease in the literary works selected here for comparison. The pandemics are occasions of "revelation" in a literal sense as the drawing back (*re*) of a veil (*velo*), but also in the sense of a *re-veiling* because the literary figure serves as a necessary cover or "integumentum" to enable us to view what is otherwise invisible. Only projection through the imagination makes this level of ultimate reality show up as observable for us at all. The imagining here works by placing numerous different registers of experience into relation with one another. Between them lies what is not itself revealed but is rather mysteriously manifest in each apparently separate domain of experience.

What is compelling about Lawrence Wright's novel *The End of October* is that it shows how the same mechanisms of contamination and corruption can be at work in different regions of the globe and even in totally disparate dimensions or aspects of reality. These transparencies demonstrate an outstanding capacity of novelistic and literary writing in general. From the tropical jungle of Indonesia, which is being destroyed by agriculture for the commercial exploitation of palm oil, to the bureaucratic stranglehold by the government's ministry of the interior blocking investigations necessary to prevent the spread of the deadly pandemic, to the social fabric of submission demonstrated by a deferential taxi driver, certain consistent overarching patterns of domination are seen or felt. The taxi driver's touchingly and courageously benevolent solicitude for his foreign client, an inspector from the World Health Organization, represents a model of what plagues society and nature alike, shown with its beguilingly benign visage. He addresses his guest as "capo," literally "head" or chief, and treats him with debonair courtesy and is even heroic in his self-sacrificing will to protect with his own life this man whom he serves as chauffer. What appears here as an inoffensively "natural" hierarchy nonetheless shows up rigid hierarchization of power as part of the injustice of the world that is at the root of ramifying problems and predations.

The End of October relates the destruction of tropical rain forests in Indonesia, terrorist attacks in Rome, a guerilla commando in Brazil, a Muslim pilgrimage in Mecca, Russian-American geopolitics, and much else besides, together with the turbulent domestic life of a family in Atlanta, Georgia. All is placed in a global network that discloses uncannily similar syndromes in each of these widely divergent spheres of activity around the world. All scenes converge upon similar patterns. A certain implicit analysis of our condition emerges from this parallel, multi-focal attention spanning such diverse sectors.

Unmistakably, plague places us before a power that we cannot master. It joins forces with a destroyer that can attack us from within since we are vowed to destruction already by our mortal nature, although we generally prefer to forget or dissimulate this ineluctable condition of our existence. Plague makes fully manifest our lack of control over life and our lack of defense against death. The recent pandemic diagnoses how completely disarmed we are to face up to such a threat and to accept our own endemic fragility despite all our technical sophistication. Like the French president Macron, we can declare war on Covid as the enemy. Indeed, there has been a worldwide call to arms against the coronavirus, but we cannot ultimately fight death as if it were an external enemy. The threat springs from within us and belongs to us as a congenital vulnerability of our physical system. It inheres in our human condition as finite and mortal.

Covid, like any plague, has forced us to the recollection of death as our final limit, as inscribed into the very shape and arc of life. There is a metaphysical dimension to this crisis that is difficult to disentangle from the merely pragmatic and technical aspects. The latter are matters that can be humanly managed to a degree. Plague, however, is the rude reminder of unsurpassable limits to our being able to ward off ultimate threats. Plague belongs to the canonical imagery of apocalypse. It has a prominent place in the biblical Book of Revelation, the Apocalypse of Saint John the Divine: "And I saw another sign in heaven, great and marvellous, seven angels having the seven last plagues; for in them is filled up the wrath of God" (15:1; cf. 16:9; 21:9). Apocalypse, too, is a virtually transparent symbol of ultimate human helplessness—but also of hopefulness in what lies beyond ourselves.[10]

---

10 Catherine Keller, *Facing Apocalypse: Climate, Democracy, and Other Last Chances* (Maryknoll, NY: Orbis, 2021), artfully ventriloquizes this ancient text, which brings the Bible to its climax, in its searing message speaking to our own times of climate crisis.

Apocalypse proclaims the end of the world as we know it. There is nothing we can do about that since all that we do is action determined from within the parameters of a given world. Both the givenness of this world and its end or destruction surpass us utterly. But therewith opens a dimension of transcendence and another kind of hope. Apocalypse, in its biblical matrix, is vitally joined with the promise of eternal life: "Be thou faithful unto death, and I will give thee the crown of life" (2:10). Eternal life serves as a prescient figure for the infinitely open dimension to which hope consigns us.

8 Theology of Hope as Negative Theology—Moltmann and Bloch

Contemplating Covid and more broadly the phenomenon of pandemic helps us to see that theologies of hope like Jürgen Moltmann's, centering on the crucified God's solidarity with suffering humans, or critical philosophies of hope like Ernst Bloch's, are most profoundly interpreted as negative theologies.[1] Bloch's work culminating in *The Principle of Hope* (*Das Prinzip Hoffnung* 1954–59) was a touchstone and became something of a foundational text for the Frankfurt school of Critical Theory. This school famously issued in some modern and even postmodern versions of negative theology in the works of Walter Benjamin and Theodor Adorno.[2] Adorno's "negative dialectics," opening Hegelian Absolute Knowing toward the Non-Identical, figures as an implicit negative theology. Benjamin's theory of the origin of "human language as such" ("die menschliche Sprache überhaupt") in the mute language of things in which their Creator speaks is overtly theological. Both thinkers touch on a register of radical alterity that implicitly entails or invites (negative) theological interpretation if we consider that negative theology consists in attempting and failing to access a relation to the absolute through means that are admittedly only relative and inadequate.

In a negative theological mode, it is by relinquishing our own determinate hopes delimited by our own conscious expectations that we can enable the salvific event to occur and bring us into its compass. This is an age-old type of wisdom powerfully expressed also in Asian religions such as Buddhism and Daoism. Their philosophies of not desiring and of not doing, or of actively doing nothing (*wu wei*), embody a wisdom that has come back into vogue from beyond and behind the overweening desire of

---

1 Ernst Bloch, *Das Prinzip Hoffnung* (Berlin, Aufbau,1954-59), 3 vols, trans. by Neville Plaice, Stephen Plaice and Paul Knight as *The Principle of Hope* (Boston: MIT Press, 1995). Jürgen Moltmann: *Theologie der Hoffnung. Untersuchungen zur Begründung und zu den Konsequenzen einer christlichen Eschatologie* (Munich: Kaiser, 1964), trans. by Daniel L. Migliore as *The Theology of Hope* (New York: Harper & Row, 1967).
2 See my *On What Cannot Be Said: Apophatic Discourses in Philosophy, Religion, Literature, and the Arts*, vol. 2, chapters 8 and 15 on Benjamin and Adorno respectively.

DOI: 10.4324/9781003545835-9

the modern *homo faber* to master everything by his own craft and technique culminating in modern technology.

Yet this negative theology is not meant to be negative in its emotional tenor. Bloch (1885-1977) was consciously aiming to reverse Heidegger's pessimistic orientation to the future through "Being-toward-death" ("Sein zum Tod") and technological apocalypse. Heidegger had labored under the spell of Oswald Spengler's theses about the decline of the West (*Der Untergang des Abendlands*, 1918).[3] Like Benjamin, Bloch was a messianic Marxist thinker of utopia, struggling to express, with a markedly Expressionist rhetoric, a horizon of hope in the midst of Germany's dark history tragically ensnared between two calamitous world wars.[4] Terry Eagleton, in *Hope without Optimism*, has more recently extended, not without sharp criticism, Bloch's reflection and this Marxist tradition of thinking about hope.[5]

Jürgen Moltmann was deliberately reacting to Bloch's renowned work in developing an explicitly theological interpretation of hope based on the doctrines of Christian eschatology as expressed in Scripture. He links the wisdom of attending to God as a higher power and lordship with a mandate for activism in the interest of social, economic, and environmental justice. The latter imperative becomes his focus in his later work to be examined later in this book (Chapter 22). Of course, the urgent need is for deep-reaching structural and systemic change in society rather than for the cosmetic changes that governments are much more willing to undertake, or at least to boast of undertaking. The *principle* of hope, as Bloch emphasizes, (re)*structures* the whole world and does not leave hope as just one more phenomenon perceived within the world.

Moltmann's "Theology of Hope," furthermore, in concert with Bloch, stresses how creative imagination works in a register of hope and how hope is the virtue orienting our life to the fullness of all its imaginable possibilities and even empowering it to attain them:

> Hope opens a wide realm for imagination and creativity. Hope makes our life dynamic, and we feel forces that we had not believed were in us. Hope makes a beginning and is the joy of anticipated fulfillment. Whoever lives in hope, sees the world no longer according to its actual

---

3 For contextualization of Bloch's philosophy, see Dr. Klaus Kufeld, director of the Ernst-Bloch-Zentrum Ernst Bloch und das Prinzip Hoffnung. - YouTube. See also Michael Löwy and Max Blechman, "Négativité et espérance," in "T. W. Adorno – Ernst Bloch," special issue of *Europe. Revue littéraire mensuelle* 86 (2008): 3–5.

4 Bloch, *Geist der Utopie* (1918, 1923), trans. by Anthony A. Nasser as *The Spirit of Utopia* (Stanford: Stanford University Press, 2000). The dark side of utopias is brought into relation with plague and apocalypse by Elana Gomel, "The Plague of Utopias: Pestilence and the Apocalyptic Body," *Twentieth Century Literature* 46/4 (2000): 405–433.

5 Terry Eagleton, *Hope without Optimism* (Charlottesville: University of Virginia Press, 2015). See Chapter 3.

reality but according to its possibilities. Higher than reality stands possibility.

Hoffnung öffnet einen weiten Raum für Imagination und Kreativität. Sie macht unser Leben lebendig und wir fühlen Kräfte, die wir uns nicht zugetraut hatten. Hoffnung macht einen Anfang und ist die Vorfreude auf die Vollendung. Wer in Hoffnung lebt, sieht die Welt nicht nur nach ihrer Wirklichkeit an, sondern auch nach Ihren Möglichkeiten. Höher als die Wirklichkeit steht die Möglichkeit![6]

This hopeful orientation has found resonance in a number of social movements of liberation. Moltmann's *Theology of Hope* (1964) has been tinder igniting a broad spectrum of liberationist projects ranging from the Black Theology of James Cone (1969), to the Latin American Liberation Theology of Gustavo Guttiérez (1971) and the Feminist Theology of Letty Russel and Rosemary Ruether (1992).[7] Negative Theology, by critically sweeping away idols, which attach absolute value to partial, relative instances, leads to and frees us for action oriented to the All and whole without invidious exclusions. As I construe it, all genuine theology is necessarily at bottom (as well as at its upper limit) negative theology since theology must acknowledge the inadequacy of human discourse to the transcendence of the divine.

Moltmann's theology of hope has been significant in sparking all of these liberationist movements as oriented to hope in the future. It belongs to the spirit of Christianity in its many forms to envisage another world different from the present one and liberated from present oppressions. Since hope in Christian theology is also eschatological and oriented toward a transcendent divinity, one that cannot be grasped or even properly be conceived by humans, a theology of hope is in a certain sense necessarily negative, at least implicitly: it aims at what is not seen but only envisaged and hoped for. As Paul's definition of hope in Romans 8:25 states: "hope that is seen is not hope." Hope's express forms need to be negated in order to turn them toward the God who transcends or exceeds human understanding and expression. Then hope can turn toward the Other that we do not comprehend in our own familiar language but need to encounter through an "apocalyptic" event, an event of revealment that exceeds our system or framework and its established forms of comprehension.

---

6 Jürgen Moltmann, "Theologie der Hoffnung im 21. Jahrhundert Vortrag von Prof. Dr. mult. em. Jürgen Moltmann Samstag, 3. August 2019, Evangelische Akademie Bad Boll Im Rahmen der Blumhardt-Gedenk-Tagung 'Damit die Schöpfung vollendet werde.'" Available online at *Microsoft Word - Beitrag Moltmann (ev-akademie-boll.de). Accessed 3-17-2023.

7 Rosemary Radford Ruether, *Gaia and God: An Ecofeminist Theology of Healing* (New York: HarperCollins, 1992). James H. Cone, *Black Theology and Black Power* (New York: Harper & Row, 1969). Gustavo Guttiérez, *Teología de la liberación. Perspectivas* (Lima: CEP, 1971), trans. Caridad Inda and John Eagleson as A Theology of Liberation: History, Politics, and Salvation (Maryknoll: Orbis, 1988; 1st ed., Maryknoll: Orbis, 1973).

9 Partial Action Combined with Hope in Wholeness

The Covid crisis provoked a flurry of frantic actions and preventative measures. The general panic resulted in an irrecusable imperative to "DO SOMETHING!" no matter what since we needed the consoling illusion that we could address and master, or at least mitigate, the problem. We desperately needed the feeling that we could be somehow remain in control and contain this threat. But the process of the pandemic revealed, instead, our helplessness. The measures taken in great haste and confusion were virtually all rescinded or abandoned not long after with similar precipitation. People could not be held back from a return to apparent normalcy once the mortal fear, but not the risk of infection, had been allayed.

So the contagion came and went and still abides, minding only its own laws of propagation and diminution. The effectiveness of every one of the measures taken remains a matter of bitter dispute and contestation among experts.[1] Africa seems to have been spared the worst in spite of its lesser preparation and presumably greater vulnerability, whereas China's apparently superior, more draconian control of the situation proved illusory, as the strict "zero tolerance" policy had to be relinquished and may even have rendered its citizens, in the end, more susceptible and defenseless.

Despite all pretention to rational scientific grounding on all sides, the only safe or face-saving *modus operandi* was imitation of others. Not knowing what to do, most did like their neighbors. Those who dared to do differently were severely criticized and often censured or ostracized. "Safety" above all, first and foremost, was everywhere on the lips of public officials and of popular pipers, as social sentiment became totally allergic

---

1 The controversy over Dr. Didier Raoult's dissenting views on the epidemic in France is a poignant illustration. To open this enormous dossier, one can begin by consulting "Controversial French doctor slams government Covid-19 response at parliament inquiry" (rfi.fr). Accessed 3-7-2023. Upholding the necessity of the measures, Jean-Pierre Dupuy, *La catastrophe ou la vie: Pensées par temps de pandémie* (Paris: Seuil, 2021), refutes the "Covid-skepticism" of leading intellectuals.

to any form of risk. Measures of whatever order are still announced and justified publicly after the motto: "For your own safety" ("Pour votre sécurité"). Debate was fierce but inconclusive—and still is. Although such information was often suppressed, serious sources tallying damages done by vaccines present them as the greater evil.[2] The general controversy and whole public debate were fraught with intractable contradictions and treacherous recriminations that could hardly be mediated by compromise or moderation.

Many, and perhaps most, prefer to see the Covid-19 comeuppance as challenging us to reinforce our ability to render ourselves invulnerable to everything. They seem to hope to overcome every obstacle to the human will to exist without the threat of death. I see it, instead, as challenging us to accept our limits and find hope therein. This is not generally what anyone wants to hear. It would not work as a platform for election of a candidate from whatever political party. In the public arena, all parties are obliged to say how they will solve all problems and guarantee ever rising levels of comfort and security and increased consumption of goods and an enhanced "standard of living." There is in my approach a frontal collision with certain accepted and consecrated values of so-called "progressive" society. Yet surely a progressive attitude might also be developed in resonance with more holistic, all-comprehensive, native perspectives on our way of being in the world. I think this outlook also resonates with certain deeper sources of thinking about hope in Western speculative traditions, which have often been anti-utopian.[3] Might our only hope lie in going back to a simpler way of living, "degrowth" (*décroissance*, as French says), rolling back some kinds of progress toward ever greater power of domination and material wealth? Might such action restore a sense of wholeness to our lives?

---

2 https://leti.lt/ybg9. Accessed 3-6-2023.

3 Johanna Jablowska, *Literatur ohne Hoffnung: die Krise der Utopie in der deutschen Gegenwartsliteratur* (Wiesbaden: Deutscher Universitätsverlag, 1993), brings this dystopian background to bear on contemporary Germanophone literature. In English Romantic literature, Mary Shelley's *The Last Man* (1826) prophesies a dystopian future set in 2070-2100 based on oracles purportedly found in the Cumaean Sibyl's cave near Naples. A pandemic of bubonic plague nearly wipes out the human race, whose governments react ineffectively.

10 Othering Hope

Postmodern, Extra-European, and Indigenous Perspectives

With the advent of postmodernity, our hopes are no longer necessarily vested in our own human projects of progressive mastery of the world. The modern expectation of steady progress without limit enters into crisis. Concerning hope, we can rejoin hands with certain pre-modern and extra-Occidental perspectives. Current philosophical reflection on hope under the banner of "apophasis" conjugates the Christian tradition of mystical apophatic theology (epitomized by Dionysius the Areopagite) with radical postmodern deconstruction (spearheaded by Jacques Derrida) in working out an approach to hope taking full account of our contemporary secular, multicultural society.[1]

Postmodern readings of Scripture emphasize the constitutive uncertainty of hope in Christian tradition—for instance, in Saint Paul's "For we are saved by hope: but hope that is seen is not hope: for who hopeth for that which he seeth?" (Romans 8:25). The postmodern deconstructive mode resonates profoundly with this apophatic religious tradition that foregrounds "the hiddenness of God."[2] Yet this hiddenness from us of a transcendent God can coincide also with an omnipresent immanence of divinity to our world and to the intimate life of consciousness that lies too close to us to be known as an object.[3]

"Apophatic" means "away from" (*apo*) "speech" (*phasis*) and designates what we cannot conceptually grasp but are inhabited and animated by, though we cannot know or say it as such. Apophasis entails a critical awareness that all our saying and knowing is already inherently a negation positing or projecting some other, prior reality as unsayable and unknowable, which it can never grasp whole. There is thus a built-in

---

1 David Newheiser, *Hope in a Secular Age: Deconstruction, Negative Theology, and the Future of Faith* (Cambridge: Cambridge University Press, 2020). My *On What Cannot Be Said*, vols. 1 and 2, lays out the broad basis of this synthesis from Neoplatonism to Postmodernism.
2 Denys Turner, *The Darkness of God: Negativity in Western Mysticism* (Cambridge: Cambridge University Press, 1999), 264.
3 See Johannes Aakjær Steenbuch, *Negative Theology: A Short Introduction* (Eugene: Cascade, 2022), 99, which concisely presents the crucial figures of this tradition.

brokenness to our linguistically mediated consciousness and the historical being it constructs.

Owning up to a certain brokenness in our history and collective being (as in our access to the divine) is first necessary to open an authentic realm of hope. Particularly indigenous experience has much to offer in the way of guiding us along this path to a hope vested not in ourselves nor in our own prowess and mastery but rather on our relationship to others and to what exists beyond us. Indigenous perspectives are usually set up in opposition to the transcendental impulses of much of Western religious culture and are typically construed as working purely through immanence, without transcendence.[4] However, transcendence need not be asserted in the form of a positive system or as the dogmatic affirmation of purported knowledge. It can, instead, be left open as a space of indeterminacy or unknowing, what we might call an "apophatic" openness.[5] So construed, transcendence turns out to be quite compatible with and even peculiarly attuned to indigenous sensibilities turned toward the mystery of the environing Great All. This attitude of openness to the Other and the All may prove to be the key to hope, I suspect, in the immemorial perspectives on the place of humans in the natural world that have been handed down by cultures now recognized as indigenous in the Americas, Australia, the Arctic, and elsewhere.

There is a form of hope that is not about optimistic expectations or rosy representations but rather about adhering to the real and simply letting it be in all its contradictory potential through resisting the impulses to delimit it with our own schemas. These restrictive impulses characteristic of our society obsessed with technological mastery and power are arguably at the root of our problem with pandemics. This posture of hope beyond hope as we conceive it is to be found among pre-Axial Age, so-called "archaic" societies. They recognize the co-implication of good and evil and do not try to reorder everything in the world in conformity with an artificially constructed transcendent ideal. Platonic Ideas, otherworldly divinities, and absolutely pure consciousness are inventions of so-called Axial-Age cultures.[6] Comprising ancient Greek philosophers and Hebrew prophets, Christian saints and Buddhist sages, Confucians and Daoists, these Axial-Age cultures have a critical side which recognizes the

---

4 A valuable guide to scholarship in this area is Fabrice Le Corguillé, *Ancrages Amérindiens: Autobiographies des Indiens d'Amérique du Nord, XVIIIe-XIXe siècles* (Rennes: Presses Universitaires de Rennes, 2021), 1–20.
5 See especially the Preface and Introduction to *Transcendence, Immanence, and Intercultural Philosophy*, edited by Nahum Brown and William Franke (London: Palgrave Macmillan, 2016).
6 Robert N. Bellah and Hans Joas, eds., *The Axial Age and its Consequences* (Cambridge, MA: The Belknap Press of Harvard University Press, 2012). See especially Charles Taylor's contribution "What Was the Axial Age Revolution?" 30–46.

transcendence of the source of all good beyond finite human grasp. But they also have a constructivist side that authorizes erection of comprehensive technological systems and totalizing institutions such as monastic orders or other organizations for managing immanent life, regulating it ritualistically in all its everyday details.

These Axial-Age civilizations proffer a utopian hope in which the negative is to be eliminated, whereas, in archaic cultures, the sacred is not cut off from the complex and immanent interweave of opposing forces in the world. The negative is lived as integral to and inextricable from the All. Good and evil are inseparable—like the ineluctable facts of eating and being eaten in the natural systems of nutrition and predation. No painstaking, thoroughgoing spiritual engineering can change that.

It is significant for our purpose that the same dialectic between traditional religious and modern scientific understandings can be found operating in Asian writings generated by experiences of plague. Although treatments are rare in Chinese literature, where plague seems to be something of a taboo subject, those narratives that do exist very clearly stage the dialectic of myth and science and even their hybridization. From the eighteenth to the twentieth centuries, various outbreaks of bubonic plague spread from Yunnan Province to the Pearl River Delta, striking Hong Kong and Guangzhou, ascending thence along the Pacific coast to northern provinces and Manchuria.

In the traditional texts that treat the subject, the Jade Emperor and his Celestial Administration, with its Department of Epidemics, were held to send plagues as punishment for the sins of the people. Stricken populations would stage public acts of contrition, begging for the intercession of deities, including Guan Yu 關羽 and Guanyin 觀音 (also known as Guanshiyin 觀世音).

The *Precious Scroll of the Rat Epidemic* (鼠瘟寶卷 *Shuwen baojuan*) by Li Shanbao 李善保, originally published in Shanghai in 1911 recounts how the bodhisattva Guanyin summoned a certain Mr. Huang Zhiren 黃志仁 in a dream to her celestial palace, Potalaka, and revealed to him that a plague was about to overrun China.[7] The bodhisattva offered to intercede with the Jade Emperor and instruct the people on how to counter the disease by repentance and moral regeneration. But she also suggested some practical measures for dealing with the plague in a way resembling modern techniques for coping with infectious diseases. Guanyin anticipated modern epidemiology with her prescient intuition that rats and fleas are the cause or carriers of the bubonic plague, and she integrates this

---

7 Li Shanbao, *The Precious Scroll of the Rat Epidemic*, trans. and ed. Wilt L. Idema, *Sino-Platonic Papers* 313 (2021), published by Department of East Asian Languages and Civilizations, University of Pennsylvania.

intuition into the dream vision with its traditional religious interpretation of the cause and dynamics of plague and its prevention.

In introducing his translation of the *Precious Scroll of the Rat Epidemic*, Wilt Idema, Professor Emeritus of Chinese Literature at Harvard University, explains that

> while Guanyin focuses on rats (and their fleas) as the carriers of the disease, she still identifies these rats as instruments of the Department of Epidemics, and while she stresses keeping cats as an effective precaution against the plague, she identifies these cats as denizens of heaven that are sent down to earth.[8]

The *Precious Scroll of the Rat Epidemic* reflects the anxiety provoked by the series of epidemics that plagued especially the closing years of the Qing dynasty (1636–1912). The plagues had been explained traditionally by Buddhist doctrine as scourges for sin, but as a modern understanding of the transmission of the disease by rats began to make headway in the nineteenth century, the two approaches were integrated. Professor Idema notes that

> Writings on epidemics are rare, and this text is interesting in combining a traditional description of the epidemics as divine punishment for the sins of humankind with more modern ideas on the cause and spread of the plague, which may have been picked up at an exhibition of public health posters.

The connection of plague with rats appeared long before there was any scientific knowledge of rats as carriers of bubonic plague. Idema quotes the "Ballad of Dying Rats" (*Shusi xing* 鼠死行) by a young poet Shi Daonan 師道南 (1772–1800), who not long after writing it became a victim of the plague. The poem clearly perceives and focuses on this natural cause yet is inscribed into a prayer calling on heaven for remission and a wish to ride to heaven on a dragon with a plea for mercy:

> Rats die to the left,
> Rats die to the right!
> When people see dying rats it is as if they see tigers:
> A few days after the rats have died,
> People die like a collapsing wall.
> —Don't ask the number

---

[8] Introduction of Wilt L. Idema to Li Shanbao's *The Precious Scroll of the Rat Epidemic*, *Sino-Platonic Papers*. 313 (2021), available online at https://medium.com/fairbank-center/plague-in-chinas-dynastic-twilight-faf6743ac8c1. Accessed 3-14-2023.

Othering Hope 57

Of those who die during the day!
The sunlight is gloomy and bleak, covered by sorrowing clouds.
Before three people have walked some ten paces or more,
Two have suddenly died and, stretched out, block the road.
—When people die at night,
One doesn't dare weep:
When plague ghosts exhale, the lamp's green flame flickers.
In a moment a storm arises and the lamp is suddenly gone:
Man and ghost, corpse and coffin share one room in darkness.
Raven caw without end,
Dogs are heard howling.
People look like ghosts:
Ghost [*sic*] steal their souls.
Most of the people you meet during the bright day are ghosts
And the ghosts you encounter after dark you take for people.
Dead people cover the ground, few houses are inhabited;
Exposed to the winds, the bones slowly, slowly decay.
There is no one to harvest the grain on the fields;
From whom can the state requisition the taxes?
Astride a heavenly dragon I want to ascend to heaven,
To call on the lord of heaven and beg heaven's mother
To sprinkle heaven's brew and dispense heaven's milk
And let it soak the soil of this world a thousand rods deep,
So all people below the earth will come back to life again
And the Yellow Sources will turn into a rain of spring.[9]

Fascinating in these Chinese texts is that the more modern scientific explanation does not simply replace the theological explanations in terms of punishment for sin sent from heaven, the way truth might be expected to wipe away myth. Instead, the two approaches are integrated as offering different, complementary, mutually supportive kinds of insight. To this day, traditional Chinese medicine works alongside Western methods and retains the trust and confidence of many modern Chinese. Might this parallel give some indication as to how native American understandings, too, could participate and serve in grasping the overall purport of plague and pandemic for our lives and our social interaction and planetary survival as a whole? Could they then help to circumscribe and reconceptualize the way Western science contributes to these questions?

Native American (Anishinaabe) writer Gerald Vizenor offers a perspective based on "survivance" as it has come to be practiced in indigenous societies. The term implies something less than overcoming

---

9 *Zhou Jinguo* 2013. Quoted in Wilt L. Idema, *Sino-Platonic Papers* 313 (2021) online: https://medium.com/fairbank-center/plague-in-chinas-dynastic-twilight-faf6743ac8c1.

opposition or conquering one's enemies, but also something more than just animal survival. For Vizenor, survivance = survival + resistance.[10] But the resistance intended here is not exactly or directly oppositional and requires a different approach from that of understanding oneself always as a victim. Vizenor's trickster character and sometime alter-ego Ronin Browne defines the term thus: "By survivance he means a vision and vital condition to endure, to outwit evil and dominance, and to deny victimry."[11] Through this character as "ironic healer," Vizenor attempts to "evade closure and victimry" (64). This approach plies indirect means of evasion for coping with a superior force that cannot be directly opposed.

Vizenor's pervasive use of "irony" is so thoroughgoing as to become, in effect, a type of apophatic discourse aligned with the "deconstructive" forms of thought that Vizenor found in Derrida, Foucault, and Baudrillard. These French postmodern theorists, who, by his own acknowledgment, deeply influenced Vizenor, model types of non-oppositional resistance that can be read as contemporary forms of negative theology or apophatic thinking.[12] I wish to think further this approach in developing my reflection on pandemics in an apophatic key as we move to contemplation of negative thinking of the unencompassable Whole to which we nevertheless in all respects and in every moment relate—or are related. Passivity and porousness are key here, hence the passive voice.

Our attempts to combat pandemics are efforts to transcend them into a condition of immunity, thereby putting an end to our vulnerability by dominating these baleful forces as foes. However, the non-oppositional approach of indigenous peoples living within the wholeness of nature and adhering to its cycles is nearer and more akin to what I would call an apophatic transcendence. This alternative is tantamount to an openness to one's environment, transcending oneself and one's own drive to know and master. It can strengthen immunity and the ability to resist through deliberate, reflective non-resistance. The not-knowing and not-saying of what masters us enables rather a fusion in which we allow ourselves to be part of the real and to be folded back into it, without eliciting and reinforcing its violence against us by struggling to master it and becoming rigid in our resistance.

---

10 See especially Vizenor's *Manifest Manners: Postindian Warriors of Survivance* (Hannover: Wesleyen University Press, 1994).
11 Gerald Vizenor, *Hiroshima Bugi: Atomu 57* (Lincoln: University of Nebraska Press, 2003), 36.
12 I work out such a connection in chapters on these figures and on Blanchot in *On What Cannot Be Said*, vol. 2, chapters 21, 24–26.

11 The Vision of the Whole versus Parceled Perception

Far be it from me to wish to make light of the coronavirus crisis or to recommend inaction in its regard. Our survival is indeed at stake. But the exclusive focus on Covid-19 as the enemy to be defeated is a false way of deceiving ourselves about the really intractable threats to our health and existence. It is a way of focusing attention hysterically on some particular and apparently tangible thing so as not to have to face the overall situation in which we find ourselves in good part because of our own doings and persistently stubborn will to continue in our suicidal penchants. The degradation of the environment, including the atmosphere, the oceans, even outer space, and the strife within ourselves and our societies issuing in destructive wars are often caused, or at least enlarged, by our increased opportunities for technological mastery of nature, time, and space, and for economic exploitation of the earth. We know all this at some subliminal level, but we are distracted by the Covid-19 crisis to embrace the illusion that we are dealing with our problems by addressing this one issue and convincing ourselves that a single technical remedy like a vaccine can resolve it.

We really know better, but this limited engagement can relieve our sense of frustration and helplessness temporarily, since we seem to be doing what we can to fight our enemy and ward off evil. The mass communications media meanwhile are doing all they can to channel our attention in just this way. And our governments, too, take measures that limit the horizon of thought and action to this immediate crisis and encourage us to forget the underlying problems and abiding threats because it seems still possible to go on a little longer along the same trajectory as in the past. This enables especially the elites who are in control of social and economic power to continue to get richer. Of course, it is a bubble that cannot last forever (like the stock market boom that has surprisingly and sinisterly accompanied the economic lockdown), an unqualified disaster for most working people and virtually all but gigantic technology-oriented companies who can exploit the exponentially increased reliance on the internet. It is all headed precipitously toward apocalypse—in the popular sense of universal destruction, at least of the world as we know it, which is to say of the world that is able to support human life and flourishing.

The more things careen out of control, the more governments and other institutions like universities tighten their restrictions on everybody, impinging thereby on productive work and on ordinary life alike. At least that way the authorities seem to be doing what is within their power to cope with the crisis. In this manner, we counter, with only a *semblance* of control, the drift toward self-destruction that hardly any government wishes seriously to confront.

An alternative approach would be to learn a lesson concerning the limits of our control and to work on transforming ourselves more into conformity with the conditions of our mortal, vulnerable, human existence that is dependent on circumambient life and on the dynamics that this life itself is summoned to respect. Changing our lifestyle to comport with ecological exigencies rather than betting on dominating enemy diseases through vaccination represents a more long-range, future-oriented response and holistic outlook. It requires us to situate Covid in the larger context of the health crisis of the whole planet.

The idea of a comprehensive "solution" that would exempt us from everything negative and ultimately from death is also a delusion to be critiqued and corrected by a perspective reinscribing us into the natural cycle in which our being, like all worldly beings, is precarious and impermanent. We can be secure, instead, not in our own being but only by being oriented beyond ourselves.

For many, the obvious implication of the Covid-19 crisis is an urgent and imperative call to action. But I am not so sure that we might not at some level actually prefer what we are in fact choosing, namely, extinction. All good things, including perhaps even life itself, have their end. This might be taken as the lesson of apocalypse. Perhaps we secretly see this as our destined end. In any case, our Faustian reflex of striving to overcome everything whatever that challenges or counters our will to power and domination (for which we resort to the magic of technology, even as Faust indentured himself to Mephistopheles and his demonic powers) can and ought itself to be mastered. Then, like Don Quixote, in Sancho's paradoxical praise of him, we could return home in defeat, but as "conquerors of ourselves" (*Don Quixote*, Part II, chapter 72). We need to overcome certain fatal impulses in ourselves in order to continue to exist—or rather to coexist with the diverse others that condition our existence and that we eliminate or suppress at our peril.

Part II
Political Ecology

12 The Web of Connections
Integral Ecology, Culture, and Society

The importance of seeing and honoring the connections between all different spheres of human life and planetary existence is poignantly stressed by Pope Francis in his 2015 encyclical *"Praised be" ("On the Care of Our Common Home")*.[1] The original title *Laudato si'* is taken literally from the *incipit* of the "Hymn to the Creator" by Saint Francis of Assisi (1181–1226). Standing as the first and incomparably majestic work of Italian literature in the vernacular, this poem celebrates the Creator through components of the Creation, starting from the sun. It is also known as the "Canticle of Brother Sun" (*Cantico del frate sole*). The verse phrase "Be praised, my Lord, for [or through] …" ("Laudato si', mi Signore, per …") is repeated at the beginning of each stanza. Using this rhetorical figure known as "anaphora," the canticle evokes *ad seriatim* the sun, the moon, fire, water, hail, frost, earth, and finally sister death. All are summoned as magnificent creations and as motives for glorifying God. The Creation in all its glory inspires reaching out in prayer to a higher, invisible, but imaginable Glory, Divinity itself.

The pope's letter to Christians and non-Christians alike, although written before the Covid-19 crisis, which broke out late in 2019 and brought the world to its knees in 2020-21, is a prescient reflection on the particularities of our situation in a globalized world of furiously accelerated exploitation of the earth's resources. The pope understands this intense activity as steeped in collective sins against the Creation that—we can now add—provoked the pandemic as only the most egregious and immediately newsworthy of myriad other catastrophes relating to the unbridled degradation and ruination of our natural environment. The encyclical already contains much clairvoyant analysis of the conditions that triggered and

---

1 Published by the Libreria Editrice Vaticana, the encyclical is available online in multiple languages at:

Laudato si' (24 maggio 2015) | Francesco (vatican.va). Accessed 3-13-2023. An English print edition exists as Francis I, *Encyclical on Climate Change and Inequality: On Care for Our Common Home*
(Brooklyn: Melville, 2015).

DOI: 10.4324/9781003545835-14

that have been exacerbated by the pandemic. Pope Francis outlines a conversion of lifestyle necessary in order to remedy a sick civilization that simply cannot be sustained. Coping with Covid becomes a matter of restoring a sane (also in the Latin sense of "healthy," *sanus*) and just relationship with the Earth and all its creatures.[2]

The pope's encyclical was saluted as "prophetic" and "eschatological" by Bruno Latour, currently France's most widely read and translated intellectual. Latour found that the encyclical marvelously reopened questions concerning "Nature" that had been closed since the seventeenth century, with the dawn of modern science. The pope penetratingly laid out the "cosmological mutation" which Latour's own later thinking circled around and endeavored to expound.[3] The pope recognized natural entities, including the earth, in their inalienable rights and in the inherent subjectivity attributed to them by Francis of Assisi's great Canticle of the Creatures. In the hymn, the creatures themselves praise their Creator in concert.

The pope's encyclical was received and reflectively transmitted in its important message for our time by a group of Italian philosophers in a collective volume applying its lessons specifically to the Covid crisis.[4] Indeed, the pandemic was experienced early and with particular acuteness and gravity in Italy. Covid-19 became a recognized national tragedy for Italy, touching even the register of the sublime, most palpably from the moment that footage of a seemingly endless convoy of military armored cars filled with coffins of coronavirus victims was aired on national public television on March 18, 2020.[5]

The pope's leading insight is that all domains of life and society need to be treated together rather than in isolation. A parceled approach comes to us almost as an automatic reflex in our age dominated, in countless concrete and practical ways, by a techno-scientific mode of thinking. But such an approach is especially insidious when applied to cases like the coronaviruses. Concentrating all our efforts on finding a medical solution, a vaccine, for a specific virus, one among tens of thousands, the one that happens to be threatening us at the moment, is shortsighted. The world turned to multinational pharmaceutical corporations such as Pfizer, AstraZeneca, Moderna, and Johnson & Johnson for salvation—companies representing just the kind of unchecked exploitation of natural resources and mass marketing strategies that lay at the root of the

---

2 For the immense Franciscan tradition behind this ecology-driven outlook and for Saint Francis of Assisi as the patron saint of ecology, see Dawn M. Nothwehr, OSF, *Franciscan Writings: Hope amid Ecological Sin and Climate Emergency* (London: T&T Clark, 2023).
3 Bruno Latour, *Qui perd la terre, perd son âme* (Paris: Balland, 2022), 16–19.
4 *L'invasione della vita: Decisioni difficili nell'epoca della pandemia*, eds. Giuseppe Civitarese, Walter Minella, Giannino Piana, and Giorgio Sandrini (Milan: Mimesis, 2020).
5 See especially Andrea Loffi, "Pandemia e sublime: Riflessioni estetiche a partire da Kant," in *L'invasione della vita*, 187–188.

problem. A much more integrated approach to reestablishing human equilibrium with the environment, as well as within society between its disproportionately privileged and its disenfranchised groups, is clearly called for in order to counter the threat. The domains of economy and culture, art and leisure are all part of the crisis that is being focused and treated by governments and media in biological and medical terms only.

The pope writes in this spirit of calling us to account for our moral stance vis-à-vis all different spheres of human life by embracing together the natural and economic and cultural facets of our collective lives. His spiritual orientation can serve as an antidote to the medicalized or otherwise purely technical approaches to crisis management or problem solving that isolate particular aspects of phenomena and ignore the underlying connectedness of all aspects and their integration with our very being as humans. As the pope writes in paragraph 111: "Seeking only technical remedies for each environmental problem that comes up means isolating things that in reality are connected and hiding the true and deeper problems of the global system" ("Cercare solamente un rimedio tecnico per ogni problema ambientale che si presenta, significa isolare cose che nella realtà sono connesse, e nascondere i veri e più profondi problemi del sistema mondiale").

After chapters on the manifestations of the crisis and on the biblical vision of Creation, the third chapter of the papal encyclical analyzes the causes of the environmental crisis as residing in an indiscriminate application of the techno-scientific paradigm of human control and exploitation of all that exists for our own utility, interests, and commercial purposes rather than finding and respecting its purpose as defined within the whole order of Creation.

Martin Heidegger's philosophy of Being stands as one of the most powerful and penetrating critiques of the technological domination of our lives that materialized in the twentieth century. Whatever judgment one adopts concerning Heidegger's compromises with the National Socialist government of Nazi Germany in the 1930s, the philosopher's thought on "the question concerning technology" remains potent and prophetic. Catholic philosopher Romano Guardini, the author of many influential works such as *The End of Modernity* (*Das Ende der Neuzeit*, 1950) and the subject of the pope's doctoral thesis, served as transmitter of the penetrating Heideggerian critique of technology, preparing the way for the pope's appropriation of it into a Catholic vision and teaching concerning human life and society.[6]

There is thus a direct line of derivation from the Heideggerian analysis of *Gestell* ("enframing"), in which every manifestation of being is

---

6 An insightful and eloquent mediator of this line of thinking to our own time and cultural situation, although expressly critical of Heidegger, can be found in Sean McGrath, *Thinking Nature: An Essay in Negative Ecology* (Edinburgh: Edinburgh University Press, 2021).

imprisoned within our human conceptualities that reduce beings to mere resources at our disposal, available for our exploitation, to Pope Francis's analysis of planetary problems in his encyclical *Laudato si'*. Concordant warnings have been issued likewise from numerous indigenous communities. Their voices have long struck this note of respect for the nonhuman and for the natural equilibrium of the Great Whole. Judith Le Blanc (Caddo), Executive Director of the Native Organizers Alliance, evokes with familiar language this consecrated outlook in an email message to her network:

> Native peoples connect with land, water, and animals of Earth not separately, but in relationship with all that is around us. We understand our role in the time continuum, past, future and present. We bring forward the ways that our ancestors best protected our Mother Earth for generations.[7]

Our astonishing, ever-enhanced technical means have increased our burden of responsibility for the environment, or the Creation, exponentially. However, at the same time, individuals are divested of responsibility. We live in a global environment that none of us individually has any power to control, although we all contribute to it, for better and worse.

Heidegger's analysis and denunciation of anthropocentric humanism as destining us to the undoing of our civilization doomed by its addiction to technological mastery and the will-to-power spoke in his own peculiar, existential language of the "forgetting of Being" ("Seinsvergessenheit"). But fundamentally the same critique emerges in innumerable other forms, including the discourse of ecology and its similarly dismal outlook on the degradation of the environment through human use and development and the excessive waste and ruin it leaves in its wake. The outbreak of pandemics is one of the many lethal consequences through which this pervasive disaster is currently and most immediately impinging on us.

For its general neglect to cultivate a contemplative dimension of its relation to the wholeness of the planet, modernity has become completely "Faustian"[8]—in the sense especially of Part II of the tragedy by Goethe, in which the protagonist becomes a tycoon entrepreneur intent on commercial exploitation of natural resources. It is left to postmodern extensions of modernity to take this totalizing refashioning of everything for one's own use and in one's own human image over the cliff to its own

---

7 More on this note by Takota Iron Eyes, Organizer of the Lakota Peoples Law Project, can be found at The UN's IPCC Report and Permanent Forum on Indigenous Issues tell us the same thing: Listen to Indigenous People! (lakotalaw.org).
8 Walter Minella, "Resilienza umana e contagio emotivo nella crisi del post-moderno," *Invasione della vita*, 96.

self-destruction.[9] The Italian philosophers analyzing our inadequacy in attempting to cope with the Covid-19 catastrophe relay the protest against this negative side of modernity in its anxious conquest of all material reality in quantitative terms at the expense of the quality of life.[10] The pope designates as "rapidación" the relentless acceleration of this reckless and irresponsible, systematic ruination. He bewails our neglect of a moral—not to say a mystical—foundation for life taken as a whole. This objection might also be formulated in ecological language akin to indigenous idioms.

---

9 I distinguish between postmodernities that continue and those that contradict modernity in "Amphibolies of the Postmodern: Hyper-Secularity or the Return of the Religious?" *Sacred and the Everyday: Comparative Approaches to Literature, Religious and Sacred*, ed. Stephen Morgan (Macau: University of Saint Joseph Academic Press, 2021), 9–33.

10 See especially Giannino Piana's opening essay "Coronavirus: L'etica provocata," to the volume *Invasione della vita*, 23–43.

13 Pandemics and Environmental Apocalypse
Their Common Causes

Is the Covid-19 pandemic a sign of impending apocalypse and of the imminent collapse of a civilization that has violated ethical norms and exceeded natural limits in the exhaustion of resources and the destruction of the equilibrium of life? There is no dearth of both scientifically documented evidence and gravely moralizing readings in this key. And there is no scarcity of macroscopic phenomena that would seem to support and even require a clear recognition of our egregious sins against one another and against our environment and fellow species as co-inhabitants of the earth.

The "Gaia hypothesis" of James Lovelock has sparked much research and speculation along these lines.[1] Lovelock initiated a discourse about Gaia, the Earth, that Bruno Latour and his followers, among many others, have embraced and developed. Lovelock writes in the Epilogue to *Gaia*:

> From a Gaian viewpoint, all attempts to rationalize a subjugated biosphere with man in charge are as doomed to failure as the similar concept of benevolent colonialism. They all assume that man is the possessor of this planet; if not the owner, then the tenant.
>
> (145)

Anne Primavesi has extended this Gaia hypothesis in explicitly theological directions, inverting the typical priority given to humanity over the earth on theological grounds. Enacting the basic move of negative theology in its essential positiveness as negation of negation and opening to infinity, she writes,

> Now after Copernicus opened the way from a closed to an infinite universe, theology can react positively by breaking open the concept of

---

1 James Lovelock, *Gaia: A New Look at Life on Earth* (Oxford: Oxford University Press, 2000 [1979]).

God: from one enclosed within a relationship with us to one unconfined and undetermined by human thought, word or action.[2]

Sean McGrath's previously cited *Thinking Nature: An Essay in Negative Ecology* stands out as a further extension and broadening of ecological thinking that is deeply inspired by negative theology. McGrath subtly thinks through the historically complex philosophical and theological roots of the environmentalist movement. More radically realizing the potential of negative thinking modeled on negative theology, he is to a certain extent building on Anthony Smith's *A Non-Philosophy of Nature*,[3] albeit with a shift in emphasis from immanence to transcendence in grappling with nature as unthinkably real. Nature's intractability to being thought and understood makes it "perverse"—after the Heraclitan motto that "nature loves to hide." Like the notion of God, the concept "nature" represents an unrepresentable whole or totality that can be approached only by negative, self-subverting strategies of thought such as have been developed exemplarily and primordially in (negative) theologies.

I emphasize that this self-critical type of thinking begins with the acknowledgment of an unfathomable divine transcendence in the Bible from Genesis and Exodus to Job and notably in the anti-idolatry critique that is so crucial to the message of the Hebrew prophets. Something of this type can be found as well in other religious traditions. Comparable accents and acknowledgments of an ineffable, divine principle transcending rational comprehension are found in the Qu'ran and in non-Western religious source texts such as the Upanishads, the Buddhist sutras, and the *Dao-de-jing*.[4]

Negative theology, particularly in its Christian incarnation, has another primal root in the natural theology of Neoplatonism. For Neoplatonism, the universe emanates from and hinges on the ineffable One-Good. The latter, however, is transcendent, inaccessible, invisible, and immaterial. Pierre Hadot, in his *History of the Idea of Nature*, interprets Heraclitus's aphorism that "nature loves to hide" in its purportedly first occurrence in an oration by the Emperor Julian in 362 CE as follows: "For Julian, it means that the gods must be spoken of in a mysterious,

---

2 Anne Primavesi, *Gaia's Gift: Earth, Ourselves and God After Copernicus* (London: Routledge, 2003), 5–6. This work stands in continuity with Primavesi's previous *From Apocalypse to Genesis: Ecology, Feminism and Christianity* (Turnbridge Wells: Burns & Oates, 1991) and *Sacrad Gaia* (London: Routledge, 2000) in denouncing the supposed theological entitlement of the human species to rule over the earth.

3 Anthony Paul Smith, *A Non-Philosophy of Nature: Ecologies of Thought* (London: Palgrave MacMillan, 2003).

4 For a comparative approach to the latter, see William Franke *Apophatic Paths from Europe to China: Regions Without Borders* (Albany: State University of New York Press, 2018).

enigmatic, and symbolic way, so that what the gods really are, their essence, may not be expressed 'in naked terms.'"[5] The Emperor Julian was transmitting fundamentally the Neoplatonic tradition, with allusions also to the Eleusinian Mysteries, the Chaldean Oracles, and the Orphic Rites. Neoplatonism represented the rational, critical, philosophical component of this highly syncretistic thinking, which was vulgarized in mythic and ritualistic forms following the refashioning and retooling of Neoplatonism particularly by Iamblichus (c. 245–c. 325), who worked in Syria, with access to ancient theologies of Egypt, Persia, Babylonia, etc. When it is recognized as contingent on divine mystery, nature can call forth critical awareness of human limitations and ignorance. The common empirical causes for pandemics and ecological crisis find here a metaphysical grounding.

In something already of a negative theological mode, Lovelock himself was well aware that our knowledge of the earth is always based on a deeper *unknowing* of something or someone who infinitely exceeds us. As he writes in the 2000 preface to his original 1979 breakthrough book *Gaia: A New Look at Life on Earth*: "This book is the story of Gaia, about getting to know her without understanding what she is" (ix). The difficulty for us is to relate to a whole beyond us and to act as responsible parts of this whole which we cannot fathom but nevertheless depend on.

> But if Gaia does exist, then we may find ourselves and all other living things to be parts and partners of a vast being who in her entirety has the power to maintain our planet as a fit and comfortable habitat for life.
>
> (1)

The ruination of soils by massive, monocultural agriculture, the strip mining of minerals, and fracking of terrains irreparably altered by extraction of their resources count among our sins against Gaia, or as the unconscionable crimes that permanently damage our environment. Our pipelines and oil barges and nuclear power plants are all prone to accidents that turn vast areas of the earth into toxic wastelands for generations to come. Our exploitation of resources knows no natural limits until something apocalyptic, something of the order of catastrophic climate change, rears its head to strike back against a species whose unchecked domination has become its own undoing, threatening humanity with its own demise. Lovelock's later work, notably *The Revenge of Gaia: Earth's*

---

5 Pierre Hadot, *The Veil of Isis: An Essay on the History of the Idea of Nature*, trans. Michael Chase (Cambridge: The Belknap Press, 2006), 71. Originally, Pierre Hadot, *Le voile d'Isis: essai sur l'histoire de l'idée de nature* (Paris: Gallimard, 2004).

Climate Crisis and the Fate of Humanity, strikes apocalyptic tones in laying out this predicament.[6]

We have drastically reduced biodiversity on the planet and encroached on the original habitats of other animal species, forcing them to adapt to living in close proximity to sprawling urban megalopolises. This proximity entails inter-species promiscuity that results in viral infections leaping across species lines that previously functioned as fire walls. Particularly wet markets in Asia, in which wild animals are kept and killed in close proximity with domesticated animals and people, have been identified as breeding grounds for new viral pandemics. Human researchers and even tourists have penetrated into the most remote reserves of wild nature, exposing themselves to untold and previously unknown microbes that are also likely candidates for starting epidemics since there are no pre-existing defenses among humans.

There is no lack of evidence that we have aggravated this susceptibility and perhaps provoked this new crisis by upsetting existing equilibriums with our methods and habits of industrial production and mass consumption. The documentation grows every day on the web and in the scientific literature based on the most diversified climatological and biosphere research conducted by institutes and researchers all around the world. Specifically, the connection between climate change and pandemics has been a frequent subject of discussion, above all in the online literature responding to the Covid-19 catastrophe.[7]

---

[6] James Lovelock, *The Revenge of Gaia: Earth's Climate Crisis and the Fate of Humanity* (New York: Basic Books, 2006). See, further, J. R. McNeill, *Something New Under the Sun: An Environmental History of the Twentieth-Century World* (New York: Norton, 2000).

[7] Coronavirus is a warning to us to mend our broken relationship with nature | Marco Lambertini, Elizabeth Maruma Mrema and Maria Neira | The Guardian. Accessed 1-5-2023. Pandemics result from destruction of nature, say UN and WHO | Coronavirus | The Guardian. Accessed 1-5-2023. See, further, Rasha Aridi, "To Prevent Future Pandemics, Protect Nature," *Smithsonian Magazine*, October 30, 2020, To Prevent Future Pandemics, Protect Nature | Smart News| Smithsonian Magazine. Accessed 1-5-2023; Damian Carrington, "World Leaders 'Ignoring' Role of Destruction of Nature in Causing Pandemics," *Guardian*, June 4, 2021, https://www.theguardian.com/world/2021/jun/04/end-destruction-of-nature-to-stop-future-pandemics-say-scientists. Numerous researchers have taken the Covid-19 crisis as requiring us to address also the issues of climate change, in particular David Klenert, Franziska Funke, Linus Mattauch, and Brian O'Callaghan, "Five Lessons from COVID-19 for Advancing Climate Change Mitigation," *Environmental and Resource Economics* 76/4 (2020): 751–778, Five Lessons from COVID-19 for Advancing Climate Change Mitigation—PubMed (nih.gov). Accessed 1-5-2023; and Krystal M. Perkins, Nora Munguia, Michael Ellenbecker, Rafael Moure-Eraso, and Luis Velasquez, "COVID-19 Pandemic Lessons to Facilitate Future Engagement in the Global Climate Crisis," *Journal of Cleaner Production* 290 (2021): COVID-19 pandemic lessons to facilitate future engagement in the global climate crisis—PMC (nih.gov). Accessed 1-5-2023.

14 Progressive versus Apocalyptic Perspectives on Pandemics

However, it is also possible to take a different view of the Covid-19 crisis with a regard turned in quite another, and even an opposite, direction. One can read this apparently colossal setback for society as a mark of progress with respect to sensitivity to the value of human life and the imperative to protect it. Pandemics are not new or unprecedented. Truly unprecedented is only the way we have reacted to this pandemic. What has most obviously and radically changed is the threshold of tolerance for accepting hecatombs of victims, especially among the most feeble and vulnerable members of society, notably the ill and aged. The Spanish flu pandemic, which raged from March 1918 to April 1920, killed more people (estimated at 50 million) than World War I, and this was generally accepted as more or less the inevitable course of things. Such resigned acceptance had previously been the norm for innumerable other decimations by infectious disease. From this perspective, the current crisis that has affected the entire world and provoked concerted countermeasures until now unthinkable might be taken to indicate a kind of advance in humanity. This would then be the opposite of an apocalyptic scenario. The progressive affirmation of human life in its infinite value could be seen to triumph in this previously inconceivable mobilization of society to defeat this "enemy."

Paradoxically, this mobilization has taken place through paralysis and has taken the form of various kinds of "lockdown." It has entailed shutting down normal life and social activity. To this extent, the presumed "advance" is riddled with biting ironies. Moreover, it is the very nature and vocation of pandemic, as I understand it, to call the idea of advance or progress into question. Plague and pandemics elicit almost inevitably the idea of apocalypse, the end of the world as we know it. Considered as apocalyptic, a pandemic arrests all progressive human development, deflating its pretensions. Apocalypse introduces a visionary perspective exceeding all our own pragmatic calculations.

An insidious consequence of our apparent progress is that we have come to expect salvation from science. The world was tremendously

DOI: 10.4324/9781003545835-16

shocked by the Covid-19 outbreak because we thought our advanced science and technology had put us out of range and risk of such lethal, life-threatening menaces as plagues. We did not expect that plague-like disease could break out among us even as in so-called backward regions of the world, just as in the Middle Ages and in Antiquity, as attested by the historical record and reflected in classic texts. The shocking aspect of Covid is its giving the lie to this false complacency and smugness. The annihilating power of the pandemic reaches to our core confidence in ourselves and in life itself. This experience, like "plague," provokes an atavistic recrudescence of primeval fear.[1]

The ostensibly augmented respect for life—in the progressive view—is bound up with a manifestly greater intolerance of the fact of death. The previously unimaginable advance in human technical capabilities for manipulating life and the environment has been accompanied by a growing inability to accept death—that is, to face our inevitable destiny as mortal creatures and perhaps even as historically conditioned societies. Have we become incapable of understanding death as intrinsic and necessary to the ongoing process of life? Do we understand human progress as infinite to the point of transcending the limit of death? How has the traditional wisdom of "know thyself" and your mortal limits become obfuscated and been forgotten in this type of ultra-modern consciousness that has found expression in "transhumanist" technologies aiming to grant the human being a kind of trans-biological immortality?[2]

Greek tragedy, with its roots in the *Iliad* and the Trojan War itself framed by a plague upon the Greek troops, was about death and even its centrality to human dignity and the sublimity of life. The Covid-19 crisis, above all, has forced us to face certain limits of our Promethean civilization in its seemingly unstoppable drive to master all reality by the power of its technological development. A kind of delayed reaction or return of the repressed has shattered our illusion of being able to continue to expand this power without limits. The pandemic has imposed a harsh and traumatizing sort of reality check. It has brought the world economy to a standstill and has arrested human productive activity in general like no other event in history.

Yet the annals of history are full of accounts of plague and pandemic, and the often surprising and paradoxical, yet predictable, human reactions prove to be remarkably consistent on analysis. A desperate denial of death and human impotence registers in the wildly disparate reactions of

---

1 Jean Delumeau, *La peur en Occident XIVe-XVIIIe siècle* (Paris: Fayard, 1978), analyzes the psychoses and traumas that result from plagues.
2 A provocative digest is found in Luc Ferry, *La révolution transhumaniste: Comment la techno-médecine et l'uberisation du monde vont bouleverser nos vies* (Paris: Plon, 2016). A penetrating critique is leveled by Olivier Rey, *Leurre et malheur du transhumanisme*.

excessive carnivalesque indulgence and promiscuity of some alongside the temperate or even ascetic responses of others. These polarly opposite reactions are carefully observed and minutely outlined by Boccaccio. Already Thucydides had noted that many, rather than being intimidated, took the plague's indiscriminate destruction as a license for indulgence and lawlessness since death would, in any case, come before any other kind of judgment (2.53). These antithetical strategies can typically be found running parallel to each other. They are complemented, furthermore, by pogroms hunting down presumably guilty parties, supposedly willful "spreaders" of contagion (as highlighted by Manzoni) to be immolated as scapegoats. All these reactions are indices of a crisis placing us before our actual lack of control of the situation.

These paradoxes are signs that the limits in question are not just objective obstacles such as the unpredictabilities of nature, which could strike fear into the heart of a peasant society, but also subjective conditions that originate from within us and from fear, at bottom, of ourselves. There is an uneasy sentiment that we are the culprits in provoking the crisis we face. This accounts for at least one side of our reaction—our turning to extreme restrictions in search of a solution. The other tendency is to trust still in "science" to provide the solution by means especially of the vaccinations touted by governments as a panacea and, in effect, salvation.

There are, at the same time, alternative expert opinions that suggest that this approach only contributes further to the underlying problems. The vaccines developed with unprecedented speed and commercialized in an atmosphere of crisis are also suspected of being potentially destructive of the delicate equilibrium on which human health and our environment depend. Some of the vaccines result in changing our genetic code with completely unforeseeable, uncontrollable consequences.[3]

The possibilities for a line of dystopic thought dwelling on the failures and fiascos of technology are legion and can be found reflected in the apocalyptic pessimism of the "Dark Ecology" movement that has taken its bearings from the works of Timothy Morton, starting from his *Ecology Without Nature* and more recently his *Hyperobjects: Philosophy and Ecology after the End of the World*.[4] The problem is no longer just with technology overtaking and suffocating being, as for the "first wave" ecological movement that found its sustenance in Martin Heidegger's philosophy and particularly in his landmark essay "The Question Concerning Technology" ("Die Frage nach der Technik," 1953, in *Vorträge und Aufsätze*). Heidegger analyzed technology as an outgrowth of the stifling

---

3 Adverse effects of drugs and vaccines in France| CMS Expert Guide. Accessed 3-6-2023.
4 Timothy Morton *Ecology Without Nature* (Cambridge: Harvard University Press, 2007); and *Hyperobjects: Philosophy and Ecology after the End of the World* (Minneapolis: University of Minnesota Press, 2013).

metaphysics that since Plato and Aristotle had destined Western thought to its tragic loss of the truly original thinking of nature as *physis* that had dawned with the pre-Socratic philosophers. A younger generation, or second-wave ecology movement, would look, instead, to technology for the solution to the environmental crisis. Yet this endeavor is paralyzed by catastrophic technological failures and impotence in the face of the immensity of our human self-undermining in the Anthropocene Age.

Morton, with his notion of "hyperobjects" is exploring the impenetrable entanglements of unsurveyable expanses and levels of reality that evade our attempts to grasp them by conventional forms of thinking. He is translating into a more scientific cultural vocabulary the kind of predicament of radical *un*knowing that, in works such as those gathered together into my *On What Cannot Be Said* (2007), has been gestated over millennia in the womb of negative theology. The outlook is somber and deeply disturbing, yet "where danger is, there grows also what saves" ("Wo aber Gefähr ist, wächst / Das Rettende auch," Friedrich Hölderlin, "Patmos").

The coming to consciousness of our limits constitutes also a condition of authentic self-awareness and effective engagement with the world. There is another kind of progress in human self-reflection to be gained from these dramatic challenges. *Memento mortis* is the traditional lesson inscribed in numerous classic artworks that have resulted from such historical calamities. Acute sensitivity to and awareness of our limits proves to be a prerequisite for the humility that is needed for a genuinely humane treatment of one another and for a responsible relation to our environment. The excruciating losses inflicted by the pandemic have also a sobering effect which calls us back to fundamental ethical principles that assert themselves anew in all their inviolability.

The humility in question entails a return to the earth or "humus" from which we come materially—and also in our etymological identity as "humans." To the earth, in the end, we must surrender ourselves: "dust thou art and to dust shalt thou return," says God to Adam in the Garden of Eden after his Fall (Genesis 3:19). This is the sobering reminder rehearsed in the Ash Wednesday liturgy of the Catholic Church. Recognition of our dependence on and responsibility to the earth, which sustains our life and reclaims our bodies in death, is exemplary of the new and acute kind of ethical-ecological consciousness fostered by the Covid-19 crisis.

This crisis serves thus as a wake-up call summoning us to undertake and effect radical changes in ourselves and in our society. We are called on to join in a collective endeavor of reconstructing the world order, building not on the foundation of the liberal individual but on networks in civil society and groupings of agents connected in pursuit of the common good. A relational concept of human being supplants, or at least expands, the atomistic understanding typical of liberal ideologies. Effective action is necessary beyond the usual moralizing about how we must change our lifestyles, our patterns of consumption, our resourcing of energy, etc. This is the spirit of the critical readings collected in the previously cited volume (*L'invasione della vita*) on the Covid-19 crisis in Italy and the world as symptomatic of a need for systemic change. Reconfiguring our relation to and position within our natural environment is the aim also of the rethinking of nature pursued by the likes of Morton, McGrath, Smith, and Lynn White.[5] The Covid-19 crisis reads as full of imperatives and instructive indications concerning the nature and means of such change.

The reflection that I offer here on pandemics and apocalypse intends to show that experiences of pandemics in cultural history have often been the occasion for visions of apocalypse in world literature. But this reflection is also meant to consider the alternatives to the apocalyptic view of the pandemic. It engages with the dialectic of views in certain exemplary cases, especially with the testimony of literary masterpieces on plagues. Although there are no prescriptions that can be applied across time from all historical instances of pandemic to our own, there is nonetheless a handing down of traditional wisdom on how to cope with this type of crisis. Filtering through classic texts, this wisdom is there to be resourced and heeded. Still, it is completely up to us to find practical ways of rediscovering and applying the wisdom of the ages in our own specific situations.

One irony is that, in all the anxiousness to return to our "normal" lives, we forget that this normalcy itself had already become dysfunctional and intolerable in many ways, perhaps even irremediably. Irresolvable tension is transformed into a nostalgically comforting image touted as "normal" only by being projected into the past in contrast to the intractable problems we face in the present and future. In this way, we miss the apocalyptic revelation that pandemic disruption offers us. To be honest, we would have to admit that we were always already at an impasse. We are constrained to learn to live in and with this impasse while at the same time striving to mitigate it. Such is the contradiction in which we contemplate our destiny through the lens of the revelatory texts of apocalyptic literature in world culture and history.

---

5 Lynn White, "The Historical Roots of Our Environmental Crisis," *Science* 155 (1967), issue 3767, March 10: 1203–1207.

15 Hope in Civil Society between Private and Public

Faced with ultimate threats and with existential challenges, citizens collaborating with one another in civil society embody a model for realizing a transcendent goal and purpose in practical ways that otherwise could not have been envisaged. Reconstruction of civil society is a project undertaken by various political movements, but also by some religious associations and academic communities.[1] In a broadly "Catholic" theological and ecumenical view, an ecological attitude is motivated by recognizing the Presence of God in Creation even while rigorously admitting the infinite distance of God from his creatures. The divine Presence is there ideally, but it needs our unreserved collaboration to be perceived and realized. By this means, the impossible can become an actual project. Changing the world, while beyond the reach of any single individual, can begin to take place in miniature in local communities. This kind of direct democratic action can be modeled, in crucial respects, also by a North American Indigenous ethos and social organization.[2]

We can employ the concept of civil society in exploring what every citizen can do to protect the environment on their own and in coordination with others acting as citizens. Our choices as consumers and as voters are the means available in our own society to change the decisions of multinational corporations and governments in the face of which the individual citizen may feel impotent. Everyone has to begin by reforming their own habits. The common citizen feels powerless when crying out in protest against government policies and industrial practices of international corporations. Popular demonstrations throughout democratic countries are blithely ignored by their governments. But the citizens' real power is in

---

1 The research group "Religión y Sociedad Civil" ("Religion and Civil Society") at the University of Navarra, led by Professor Montserrat Herrero, in which I have been privileged to participate since 2019, has been a model matrix of such community for me personally.
2 Path markers include Bruce Johansen, *Forgotten Founders: How the American Indian Helped Shape Democracy* (Boston: Harvard Common Press, 1982); and Vine Deloria, Jr., *God Is Red: A Native View of Religion* (New York: Putnam, 1973), 203–218.

DOI: 10.4324/9781003545835-17

changing their own lives and then sharing their approach and amplifying it by association with other like-minded individuals or groups, for example, by boycotting products that are damaging to the general good and by adopting alternative lifestyles that are more conservation-friendly. This is how society can be changed by human beings acting on their consciences more than by systems of governance that are typically bound by conservative inertia and beholden to vested interests of political and economic privilege.

Civil society consists not just in independent individuals vying with one another for advantage and thereby supposedly serving the common good in spite of their own selfish intents, as in the classic liberal theory of Adam Smith, with its emblematic "invisible hand" of providence. Instead, the members of civil society understand themselves, in their core and origin, not just as separate individuals but rather as existing in and with and from their common bond. An organic community is the model of society that can be found in various forms among indigenous peoples and in archaic civilizations, and these models can serve today to guide our transition to alternative forms of social organization and networking.

We find in these models the ethos that inhabits the human community long before it is formalized into the institutions of the State. In the interstices between public and private spheres, civil society constructs the tissue of common life from which both of these poles inevitably proceed and to which they are oriented. Times of crisis, like war and pandemic, have been exemplary historically in bringing to the fore this otherwise often hidden fabric of society—along with its opposite, the *un*civil society that breaks out with the break-down of the State and the breaking-up of respect for anything such as a private realm as well. Violations of rights and liberties, through the arrogation of extraordinary and undemocratic powers to the State operating in a state of emergency, are the common lot and liability of pandemics. This consolidation and bearing down of State power is perfectly compatible with, and may even be provoked by, the State's being threatened, at the same time, with disintegration.

"Lockdown" is a form of reaction that unwittingly images the paralysis and consternation induced by confrontation with the uncontrollable threat represented by plague or pandemic. Just as, in the past, plague served as a call to conscience and as a stimulus for correcting one's life, still today the pandemic reminds us searingly that we always can and need to seek more socially and ecologically just ways of living. Imperative for this purpose is an expanded consciousness reaching beyond our usual conceptual thinking geared to definable entities.

16 From Social to Cosmic Consciousness
Latour's Apocalyptic Reading of the Coronavirus Crisis

Cultivating an attitude of peaceful coexistence can, and perhaps must, extend far beyond the parameters of society into cosmic consciousness. It entails an unspecialized, open, contemplative regard on Being and Creation that does not see the world in purely pragmatic terms as a resource to be exploited but rather as a living organism to which we are summoned to adapt and submit ourselves. This attitude is commonly held to be characteristic of indigenous approaches, notably in native North American cultures, and it is also taken up by a wide spectrum of ecologically minded currents of critical thinking promoted by modern or postmodern Western philosophers. Bruno Latour's critique of modernity and its nature-culture dichotomy is among the most widely recognized sources of such reflections emerging in the discipline of philosophy.[1] These newly accentuated representations of the earth feature centrally also in the discourse of numerous sorts of environmental activism.

Latour, however, tries to wean thought away from myths of the earth as a pagan goddess, the Great Mother, and even from concepts of it as Globe and as Nature. Earth, instead, is constituted by the concerted and conflicted activities of living and non-living things: it stands as the interactive background of our actions. Latour's is rather a negative way of thinking the power that stands over us and impinges on us in an imperious, unignorable manner that nevertheless depends on how we ourselves act and impinge on it in an influence loop. Thus, the earth cannot quite be totalized in a concept that would lend itself to mythologization. It is experienced, instead, in pragmatic interaction.

---

1 See particularly Bruno Latour, *Face à Gaia: Huit conférences sur le nouveau régime climatique* (Paris: La Découverte, 2015), trans. Catherine Porter as *Facing Gaia: Eight Lectures on the New Climatic Regime*. (Cambridge, United Kingdom: Polity Press, 2017). The first chapter is on the instability of the notion of "nature." See also Bruno Latour, *Où atterrir? – Comment s'orienter en politique* (Paris: La Découverte, 2017), trans. *Down to Earth: Politics in the New Climatic Regime* (Cambridge: Polity Press, 2018).

This approach coincides with what I interpret as the anti-idolatry polemic of negative theology, which I am here applying to the analysis of pandemics. It resists static, determinate concepts and images of God or goddesses. Yet recognizing the Earth as alive and intelligent in ways surpassing our own living and knowing is as important to Latour as is theism (affirming a personal God) to theology. We simply need to retain a critical awareness of the negativity and inadequacy of all our conceptions of such realities since the realities surpass us even as they enable and sustain our very ability to think about them. Latour converges on an at least secular theology, furthermore, in viewing the environmental crisis as apocalyptic, as a revelation of an irrecusable challenge to our survival and salvation.

Latour interprets the coronavirus pandemic as symptomatic and as preparing us for the tremendous trials of coping with human-induced climate change.[2] The Covid-19 experience was a concentrate of all that lies before us in our now disturbed relation with our environment and, even more comprehensively and momentously, with the Earth. Before he died on October 9, 2022, Latour reflected in his final work dealing with the confinement induced by the coronavirus pandemic as epitomizing our confinement on Earth. This confinement is popularly rehearsed in the slogan: "there is no planet B." It reveals our predicament and can constrain us to correct our mode of being on the earth. It occurs now as an apocalyptic event ushering in a new era for humanity and the earth. Latour baptized the result of this birth: "the New Climate Regime" ("le Nouveau Régime Climatique"), which would be decisive for our survival and for that of millions of other species as well.[3]

The rhetoric of war was mobilized by French president Emmanuel Macron and by other leaders in addressing their nations with the summons to rally to the defense of their very lives in fighting against the virus.[4] Fighting against viruses, however, is in some degree contradictory inasmuch as we are constituted by viruses, among other things, and have integrated them always already into our own biological system. We cannot completely eliminate viruses without eliminating ourselves.[5] Some kind of

---

2 Bruno Latour: "Ce virus est là pour nous préparer à l'épreuve suivante, le nouveau régime climatique" | France Culture (radiofrance.fr). Accessed 7-7-2021.

3 Latour, *Où suis-je? – Leçons du confinement à l'usage des terrestres* (Paris: La découverte, 2021).

4 "'Nous sommes en guerre': face au coronavirus, Emmanuel Macron sonne la 'mobilisation générale,'" *Le Monde*, March 17, 2020, available online at: https://www.lemonde.fr/politique/article/2020/03/17/nous-sommes-en-guerre-face-au-coronavirus-emmanuel-macron-sonne-la-mobilisation-generale_6033338_823448.html. The next day President Donald Trump tweeted: "The world is at war with a hidden enemy. WE WILL WIN." https://twitter.com/realdonaldtrump/status/1239997820242923521. Accessed 4/19/2023.

5 Thomas Pradeu, *The Limits of the Self: Immunology and Biological Identity*, trans. Elizabeth Vitanza (Oxford: Oxford University Press, 2012), shows scientifically the artificiality of dichotomizing between self and non-self. He pursues the speculative implications in Thomas Pradeu, *Philosophy of Immunology* (Cambridge: Cambridge University Press, 2020).

symbiosis has to be sought that would balance the claims of harmonizing with the whole and defending one's own particular niche and charter for existence as a specific life-form or species. For species, like individuals, vie with one another for the resources necessary for life.

One sees the trees striving upward for light in a forest and alongside them the unlucky fate of other plant species living in the shadow or condemned to extinction for lack of the ability to secure their required share of light. Our identity as humans needs to mediate between our being one specific life-form and our conscious awareness of the All of which we are a part. Yet perhaps the particulars of this human "we" are fluid in form and need not be strictly identified with any achieved organism or static and essentialized species type. We can give ourselves up in certain familiar, achieved forms for the sake of facilitating transformation into other possibilities of existence.

We are part of the fight to survive, but we can also look out beyond it and holistically affirm the goodness of the whole—echoing the biblical Creation account in Genesis 1: "And God saw that it was good"—in which all particular forms are destined to perish in time. These metaphysical perspectives I deem to be useful in order to help us keep in perspective our own needs and desires, our anxieties and ambitions. At some psychological level, we can live in peace while defending our interests and existence against encroachment from invaders, as any species must do if it is going to survive. We might even, in this regard, recognize our kinship with many predator species who need to kill in order to eat. The sovereign calm of the lion, even in distress during drought and dearth of prey, becomes pertinent as a tragic moral emblem for us.

However, we are not bound by necessity in exactly the same way as are other animal species. We can also transcend the condition of relative savagery observable in nature through our reflective consciousness. The difference between dwelling in universal harmony and living embroiled in the war of all against all is, first of all, one of perspective. And each different perspective may be valid in its own proper sphere of application. Our identity articulates itself differently at these different levels of perception, individual or collective. Can we choose to give ourselves the benefit of a benevolent outlook on creation, embracing all species in fraternal-sororal amity? Such is the enrapturing lyrical vision of Saint Francis's "Canticle of Brother Sun." This attitude requires learning a certain detachment from an ideology based on control of nature through scientific knowledge—as expressed emblematically in Descartes's founding charter of modern science and its promise to make us "masters and possessors of nature" ("maîtres et possesseurs de la nature" *Discours de la méthode*, 1637).

17 Relativizing Scientific "Truth"

There are many different methodologies and different sciences answering to diverse exigencies in our array of specialized knowledges. And many errors have been made in the scientific evaluations of Covid-19 (SARS-CoV-2-WIV) and in society's defense against it.[1] Pandemic and the panic it lets loose upon the world seem to be custom-made for prompting all manner of hysterical distortion and misrepresentation and for engendering false "facts." The word "*pan*dem*ic*" itself tends by its anagrammatical suggestions to disseminate panic. The contradictions and controversies about simple procedures such as wearing masks, social distancing, disinfecting gels, and other sanitary protocols, not to mention vaccinations, proliferate because reality itself is never as simple as we make it out to be. Clinical and everyday applications are never quite as easy and straightforward as laboratory science. Moreover, because of the crisis situation with Covid-19, scientists have been under considerable societal pressure to produce simple answers and easy-to-implement solutions. Of course, we know that science is also often corrupted by economic influences since laboratories operate in fealty to large corporate structures that can sometimes work at cross-purposes to the public interest because of being driven by profit.

We heard every day, with a degree of disbelief, at over a year from the first "lockdowns" being implemented and still reimplemented, that the virus was still not under control despite the draconian measures adopted. We were told that we had to submit to more and more stringent requirements and restrictions on public and even on private life. The media admitted with astonishment, and most of us never imagined, that after a year the whole world would still be struggling in such a manner to recover from the devastating effects of the pandemic. We all seemed to have forgotten that the security and hygienic measures imposed by the government were designed only to *slow down* the spread of the virus. That was

---

1 Giorgio Sandrini, "Scienze e società: Tra verità e post-verità," in *L'invasione della vita*, 45–76.

DOI: 10.4324/9781003545835-19

what we had done and were still endeavoring to do, at least according to the logic of the measures taken. We seemed to have turned this health crisis into an ongoing and even permanent change to our whole way of life in attempting to do just the opposite. We imposed supposedly temporary emergency measures for what is really a chronic problem in our relation to the earth and reality.

Bruno Latour argues that the "enemy" is among us and even within us. He articulates this more complex vision of the presence of viruses as constitutive of the fabric of life and as contributing to producing the conditions necessary for life on the planet.[2] Latour's thinking about the sanitary crisis is extended in the terms of his late thinking centered on the earth or *Gaia* as revealing to us our condition as terrestrial beings existing in interdependence with the totality of beings. This reciprocity cannot as such be hypostatized. It evades the objectivizing mode of thought typical of the positive sciences.

Latour also reconfigures science as ensconced in society and as steered by certain cultural myths rather than as an exceptional form of knowledge overcoming all myths. In radio emissions on *France Culture*, he addresses these issues as they are raised specifically by the Covid-19 crisis.[3] Following up in this vein, Patrice Maniglier's lucid development and application of Latour's "terrestrial" thinking focuses exclusively on how it explicates the Covid-19 pandemic and vice versa.[4]

Maniglier emphasizes how Latour's work makes us realize that science does not deliver answers but opens new questions and problems. Science "brought down to earth" consists concretely in controversies and disputes. People began to take notice of this contentious character of science when the Covid-19 crisis and its pervasive impingement on everyone's lives made a larger, lay public interested enough to look into the alternative scientific theories and hypotheses and realize how up for grabs scientific theses really are. None are infallible or indisputable. Science is presented by Latour as a battlefield where each theory competes for the maximum number of adherents. This battle is based on relations of force. Numbers of allies and their weight as authorities determine which theory wins (Maniglier, chapter 1). For Latour, this battle scene offers a more realistic understanding of how sciences actually work but does not undermine their authority. I agree that Latour gives a more realistic understanding of how scientific authority is actually constructed, but he leaves us with the

---

2 Bruno Latour, *Pasteur: Guerre et paix des microbes*, suivi de *Irréductions* (Paris: La Découverte, 2001).
3 Bruno Latour: "Ce virus est là pour nous préparer à l'épreuve suivante, le nouveau régime climatique" | France Culture (radiofrance.fr). Accessed 7-7-2021.
4 Patrice Maniglier, *Le philosophe, la terre et le virus: Bruno Latour expliqué par l'actualité* (Paris: Broché, 2021).

problem that minority views can often be more true and accurate than those subscribed to by the many and by more powerful parties and elites. Allies are assembled by means of persuasion and by pressures of power having nothing to do with the intrinsic truth of the theory or with the validity of the cause in question.

    I believe that Latour's point cannot be simply that "might makes right" but rather that there is no other way for the right answers and analyses to emerge and prove themselves except by the continual process of debate and the attempt to persuade others, which can and often does involve various types of forcing. Bringing science down to earth and into the world leaves no other superior court of appeal to adjudicate its disputes. Latour's thinking is thus rightly ranged under the sign of immanence. And yet neither can it be correctly or categorically opposed to all types of transcendence whatever. For the fact of debate to make sense at all there must be a possibility of appealing to truth as the final goal and arbiter, even if it can never be accessed as such but only through the interpretations of mutually contesting participants in debate. All contenders maintain not simply that they are the stronger party but that their position on some scientific question is more correct and portrays how things really are.

18 Truth and Transcendence versus Technique

We might easily be persuaded by such an earth-oriented philosophy as Latour's into thinking that a sane approach to our earth must exclude all thinking of a transcendent divinity as a kind of arch-error or original sin of Western philosophical thinking. Worship of such an abstraction of transcendent divinity might seem logically to lead to disrespect of the earth and its creatures in their immanent presence. Hence renouncing all ideals and conceptions of the transcendent would be called for to cure our sick Western (in)disposition. A further inference might be that by rejecting any form of transcendence we come closer to the native American Indian or Indigenous attitudes that are naturally conservationist. This, however, I think, is a mistake and gives only a facile illusion of overcoming the problem that has led to our current impasse. To truly understand something of the deeply spiritual outlook of many Indigenous peoples, we do better to dig deep into our own spiritual traditions of mystical love and apophaticism. They have all along adumbrated a radical alternative to the pure pragmatism of our more typically modern, Western, empiricist approaches to inhabiting the planet.

It is not exactly the orientation to an ideal or transcendent truth that is responsible for miscarriages of our dealings with the earth. Only when this transcendence is fixed in concrete and idolatrous terms does it become deleterious. What we should fear more than orientation to an indeterminate transcendence is the reductively empirical and managerial pragmatism of dominant strains of Western culture. Despite all due acknowledgment of the amazing accomplishments of our human technology, taken on its own it leads us into a cul-de-sac. Heidegger's critique of the technological norming of our culture, ensconced within his philosophy of finitude and immanence, adhering to everyday experience rather than to metaphysical formulas, is based on human *being-there* or "Da-sein" as constantly transcending itself, as suspended in the temporal ecstasies toward past and future that make *Dasein* constantly reach out beyond its given present.

DOI: 10.4324/9781003545835-20

Given the differential logic of language and concepts, there are certain forms of transcendence that are immanent, that belong to immanence itself. Any *thing* declared to be transcendent in itself, any *separative* transcendence, is suspect and indeed idolatrous. Yet self-transcendence, transcending oneself into or toward others to whom one is intrinsically related, has to be constitutive of any earth-bound ontology. An apophatic transcendence that holds open and acknowledges an undefined space for what exceeds any given object and act of knowing as its condition and ground is finally, I submit, very much in the spirit of Latour's own turn of thinking.[1] Only our ends and purposes can steer our reception of the truth that counts for us, yet this sovereign truth, which Latour recognizes as "Gaia," imposes its conditions on us without repeal. This is not a truth formulated in words but a presence-absence that is an absolute for us, one that we must honor and acknowledge by obeying its imperatives. Such a revolution in the conception of truth can be heard also in the Christic declaration "I am the way, the truth, and the life" (John 14:6). This declaration expresses a personal reality that cannot be mastered by any technical means.

We have developed remarkable technical efficacy. We have invented prodigious means, but we have failed on the whole in discerning what commonly beneficial ends are actually worth pursuing. Science does not answer this question for us. It furnishes means but does not decide ends. It ascertains facts, not values (*pace* Sam Harris), although Latour has shown that science, far from being purely descriptive, intervenes actively in constructing the reality we imagine and inhabit.

Latour's sociology of science has stressed that it is just one among many forms of knowledge and is subject, like the others, to social norms: it is not some kind of superior or absolute truth. The ethos of modernity has often been based on a confidence in science as an exceptional kind of knowledge and as exempt from subjective interpretation and political conditioning, but this view is refuted by a more adequate knowledge of the history and sociology of science. Such knowledge is prerequisite to the rethinking of the politics of science that lies at the ground of Latour's thought and forms a basis for the critique of the coronavirus politics that his thought has delivered and stimulated.

---

[1] "Apophatic" or indefinable transcendence is explicated in *Transcendence, Immanence, and Intercultural Philosophy*, edited by Nahum Brown and William Franke (London: Palgrave Macmillan, 2016), beginning with the Introduction.

19 Negative Theology of the Earth According to Bruno Latour

Certainly, "immanence" is the watchword of Latour's philosophy and of the entire ecology movement. We need to focus our concern on this concretely present earth and not on some other world. Yet the Earth exists only in its "translations." As Maniglier explains in expounding Latour's thought, the Earth cannot be grasped except through the events in which it manifests its function of "localizing the global" ("'localizer le global'... on ne peut saisir la Terre qu'en la reconduisant à chacun de ces événements où elle manifeste sa fonction de *localisateur*").[1] This means, after all, that the Earth has a kind of transcendence with respect to any of its concrete manifestations—despite Maniglier's determination to "exorcise every risk of transcendence" ("conjurant tout risque de transcendance," 141).

There is an ontological difference between the earth and everything that happens on it, and this makes for a kind of transcendence of the Earth. Earth is not reducible to phenomena measurable by our earth sciences. The problem is not with transcendence as such, but with treating worldly entities as transcendent. Theologically considered, such treatment is idolatry. What is truly transcendent is never a thing that can be grasped but the vital force that animates us and everything else on the earth. We might recognize this life force as the Earth herself and indeed as transcendent of all our science. Latour, in fact, distances himself from ecology and its modes of thinking because they pretend to reduce all reality to the measure of our human calculations.

Latour's work resituates science, placing it back into the world rather than allowing science and human subjectivity to hover above and transcend the world. Stripping science of any transcendent airs restores the truly transcendent beyond our science and our knowing. Transcendence reappears as the life force that animates us and even grants us our existence.

---

1 Maniglier, *Le philosophe, la terre et le virus*, 136.

Latour recognizes that relating to Gaia entails a theology[2]—and a thanatology. He also intuits the inherently negative nature of this theology—as of all authentic theology, I might add. Theology thought through to its ground in what no finite formula can grasp is inherently negative. Latour's Earth, as the negation of its many manifestations, repeats the logic of the transcendent God of negative theology, the God with many Names, none of which can be more than heuristic.[3]

Making constant reference to the pope's encyclical *Laudato si'*, Latour outlines a penetrating understanding of how some form of transcendence is always folded into immanence. This ineluctable type of transcendence is found in what we might call relational thinking. Nothing can be fully understood except as it relates to everything else. Any thing's being transcends it into every other being. "This world of living things is as 'transcendent' as possible in this very concrete sense that their interactions constantly 'surpass' them" ("Ce monde des vivants est aussi 'transcendant' que possible en ce sens très concret que leurs interactions se 'dépassent' constamment elles-mêmes," 62). Latour shows himself here to be sensitive to the existential logic of transcendence that has been thought throughout the ages in its mind-boggling intricacies by the immense resources of theology as it has been experienced and lived out in religion. He confesses himself to be inspired throughout his whole life in particular by Catholicism ("inspiré depuis toujours par le catholicisme," 45).

The living system of interrelations that make up the Earth as a whole cannot be totalized as a thing. It transcends every reductive definition by concepts because it is alive and dynamic, the living (and dying) Earth. For Latour, the new cosmological view, in which we are confined to the earth, requires something like a religious conversion to be accepted and comprehended, or even just perceived as possible (41). He laments the difficulty he has in "transmitting" this awareness to his friends and colleagues, with their "lay" ("laïque," secular) culture closed to the prophetic and apocalyptic horizon of the pope's message (42, 45). Latour recognizes in theology one of the different and incommensurable modes of truth that make sense in different dimensions of existence. This "religious truth" ("verité religieuse," 43) can now be appreciated in its just measure non-hegemonically.

---

2 See especially Latour's engagement with theology from beginning to end of *Qui perd la terre, perd son âme* (Paris: Balland, 2022), trans. Catherine Porter and Sam Ferguson as *If We Lose the Earth We Lose our Soul* (Cambridge, UK: Polity, 2024). Parenthetical page references to Latour's writing in this chapter and the following Chapter 20 are to the French edition of this work. English translations are my own.

3 In just this vein, Eduardo Viveirso de Castro and Déborah Danowski directed a conference on "The Thousand Names of Gaia" at Rio de Janeiro in September 2014. See Déborah Danowski and Eduardo Viveirso de Castro, eds., *The Ends of the World* (Cambridge: Polity Press, 2017).

Negative Theology of the Earth According to Bruno Latour

Speaking of the mode of truth of theology, we must remember that theology is always at its root and ground *negative* theology because divinity transcends human grasp and understanding, every *logos*. In the end, divinity can be expressly understood only self-reflexively as a product of human reflexivity since it is the nature of *theos* to transcend all worldly being and understanding. The *discourse* of theology always has to negate *itself* in order to gesture toward its true intent and meaning, which is divinity beyond speech: it is present like "Gaia" so concretely as to grasp *us*, even before we can begin to try to grasp *it*. The space of the earth, particularly the "critical zone" of the living between soil and atmosphere, is the dimension that grasps us and holds us in life beyond and before all our conceptions and ability to conceive and comprehend it. It will decide whether we live or die, no matter how we conceive of it. It transcends our willing and conceiving.

This "critical zone" may well be an immanent transcendence, but then, symmetrically, it also implies or enfolds a certain transcendence of immanence. Immanence absolutized transcends any inner-worldly thing that we can understand—we cannot "stand under" or get outside of it. *Gaia* has a kind of reality transcending human grasp and language. The use of the Greek word for the earth as a proper name indicates this ineffable transcendence, as Latour points out.[4] Proper names do not properly belong to language; they have no proper meaning (sense) but only a denotative function (reference).[5] They designate the unique essence of an individual being which transcends expression in language (*individuum ineffabilis est*).[6]

This unique reality is fundamentally unknowable, but recognizing its existence is essential to keeping knowledge open to the whole that it cannot encompass and cannot as such know. We encounter something in principle unknowable in every domain of knowledge as the underlying object around which all knowledge revolves yet never grasps or exhausts. The imperative of an impossible wholeness is what keeps knowledge open to the real and presents it from reducing to a closed, merely self-referential system.

---

4 Latour, *Où suis-je? – Leçons du confinement à l'usage des terrestres* (Paris: La découverte, 2021), 39–52, chapter 4: "'Terre'" est un nom féminin, 'Univers' est un nom masculin," especially 47–52.
5 Gottlob Frege, "Über Sinn und Bedeutung," *Zeitschrift für Philosophie und philosophische Kritik* 100 (1892): 25–50, trans. M. Black as "Sense and Reference," *The Philosophical Review* 57(1948): 207–23; cf. Bertrand Russell, "On Denoting," *Mind* vol. 14, no. 56 (1905): 479–493.
6 Cf. Franz Rosenzweig, *Der Stern der Erlösung*, ed. Albert Raffelt (Freiburg im Breisgau: Universitätsbibliothek, 2002), 207–208, trans. William W. Hallo as *The Star of Redemption* (Boston: Beacon Press, 1964).

Part III
Apocalyptic Hope

20 Eschatology, Incarnation, Kenosis

The limits of the earth are eschatological and will decide, beyond our capacity to deny or resist, whether we live or die. Eschatology, as reconceived in Latour's New Climate Regime, concerns not a distant future to be imagined and expected but our immediate living space. The current apocalyptic situation of our critical space for living contains a call to immediate action: do or die.[1] Only by acknowledging this sovereignty of the Earth, which we cannot live without, can we focus on the necessity of acting so as not to destroy it. Earth's sovereignty means that it is not just a resource for our use but a Giver and Sustainer of life who we must obey or else .... We wish to impose our own will and understanding on it, but in reality Earth's dispositions have sovereign power over us.

Negative theology thinks always from the limits of what is thought and of thinking itself. Latour's philosophy conduces to a negative theology of the Earth by thinking the limits of our earth and of our earth science. His thinking enjoins acting to safeguard the "critical zone" or the envelope of the biosphere that grants species life and enables life to survive.[2] Latour develops this thinking with various figures for the Earth that he recognizes as theological in tenor. Yet, as negative theology insists, all theological concepts are necessarily figures since no proper knowledge of God is possible for humans, at least not in purely natural terms. Revelation of God is conceived of by Church doctrine as miraculous, as exceeding what is naturally and humanly possible. Negative theology radicalizes this insight by stressing that God is humanly unsayable and even inconceivable. A negative theology of the Earth begins from the insight that there are limits to our ability to think and understand the Earth.

1 Latour acknowledges a fundamental debt for his analysis to Isabelle Stengers's apocalyptic outcry in *Aux temps des catastrophes: résister à la barbarie qui vient* (Paris: La Découverte, 2009).
2 Bruno Latour and Peter Weibel, eds., *Critical Zones: The Science and Politics of Landing on Earth* (Boston: ZKM and MIT Press, 2020) leverages a 2020 exhibition at the Center for Art and Media Karlsruhe (ZKM), deploying visual and literary arts to contemplate the changing landscape in which modern humans live.

DOI: 10.4324/9781003545835-23

Latour employs certain key negative theological concepts, notably salvation and *kenosis* understood as an extension of *incarnation*: "The ecology crisis *extends* in the same direction that incarnation had already indicated. Salvation lies in the direction of abasement, kenosis" ("La crise écologique *prolonge* la direction même que l'incarnation désignait déjà. Le salut est vers l'abaissement, la kénose," *Qui perd la terre, perd son âme*, 62). Latour is thinking the limits of anthropocentrism in our Anthropocene age and finding there a kind of negative theology that pivots on a kenosis (literally "self-emptying") of abasement through incarnation—Christ's humbling himself to become flesh. This movement downward to earth is "kenotic" as modeled on Christ, who, though being of the very nature and essence of God, emptied himself and accepted embodiment as a man and even humiliation and death on the cross, as celebrated in the hymn of the Pauline Epistle to the Philippians 2:5-12. Kenosis is a downward movement grounding itself in the immanent. Kenosis entails surrender of transcendent divinity in accepting incarnation as human and so is an immanentization. Nonetheless, this remains an act of transcendent divinity.

Theology of incarnation as kenosis is a negative theology, negating our conventional notions of divinity as impassive, eternal, all-powerful, etc. The humiliation and self-emptying of Christ reveals God as a God of infinite love for his creatures and willingness to suffer and even die for their redemption. This gesture embodies and enacts the living and dying for one another that characterizes what takes place throughout the Creation itself. The dependence of humanity on its Creator has revealed itself concretely as a dependence on the living creatures that have indeed created the biosphere which enables humans to live. Our salvation depends on its preservation.

Latour recognizes the antecedence and preeminence of the "autochthonous" or of indigenous peoples in the art of caring for the world (65). Nevertheless, he introduces some important nuances with respect to most traditional conceptions. His own vision is not so much of Earth as a mythological person whom we offend, or as a hyper-organism whose harmony we disturb, as of a network of interactive beings all continuously acting on and reacting to one another.

The figure of Earth as a simple unity is negated as much as *theos* is by this process of mutually constitutive inter(re)actions among all living things. Yet there is something about this ongoing interchange that still invites symbolization in terms of transcendence and unity and, to that extent, as divine. This model should not be understood as reducing all to mere chemical-biological processes but rather as opening the density of material process to its incomprehensible depth and spiritual mystery. All the complex entangled relations of creatures are hosted on *one* Earth. This transcendent being cannot exactly be accessed and described as such nor be identified with the globe or with any other purely immanent entity.

Nevertheless, the unity of all living things in their mutual dependence is circumscribed by the Earth as the indispensable Creator and Sustainer of the life of all. That the Earth is *one*, for Latour, cannot be grasped conceptually. Instead, this oneness is experienced and constituted concretely through participation in the interconnected continuity of finite living beings in their totality.[3]

A negative theology of the earth is one that is directed downward, toward the earth, intent on landing (*atterrir*, etymologically "earthing") rather than looking up to heaven for escape.[4] Salvation can come only from caring for the earth, which is the source that has created the heaven or the atmosphere that surrounds the earth through the exhalations of living creatures starting from primeval bacteria.[5] Earth and its creatures are recognized as the life-giving, creative source of "heaven" (the sky, the atmosphere) in the New Climate Regime, which Latour prophetically declares as operational for our post-Covid Age. Acknowledging the prophetic lead of Pope Francis, Latour underlines that this new theology of the earth is "apocalyptic" (92ff). At stake is precisely the end of the world—but in the sense also of the end or goal to be pursued and fostered (co-existence rather than domination)—as well as the threat of imminent extinction.

Against his strongly secularist friends and associates, who are intolerant of religion and its symbols and figures, Latour recounts attempting in vain to explain the new pertinence of Christian eschatology to our current crisis. Necessary here is the work of preaching and conversion in a domain of persuasion. In contrast with civil religions and cosmic religions, which attempt to endure and to discipline and dominate time, Latour's religious vision envisages the "irruption of a time that does not pass into time that passes" ("dans le temps qui passe, fait irruption un temps qui ne passe pas," 95). This time (or eternity, unpassing time) is paradoxical and requires always new figures in order to begin always anew to be understood.

Referring to Jan Assman's theory of counter-religion, Latour contrasts the new (monotheistic) religions of rupture and liberation with the old civic and cosmic religions concerned rather with assuring continuity. From this revolution (which I previously treated as the Axial-Age shift in *On the Universality of What Is Not*, chapter 8) comes an orientation of religion to a higher reality looking away from the earth. A rift between what judges and what is judged also rives asunder the cosmic whole.

---

3 Maniglier, 66–71, elaborates the "axis of continuity" as crucial to Latour's thought. Mauro Ceruti and Francesco Bellusci, *Umanizzare la modernità: Un modo nuovo di pensare il futuro* (Milan: Cortina, 2023) develop a related approach to thinking this interconnectivity of all.
4 Bruno Latour, *Où atterrir? – Comment s'orienter en politique* (Paris: La Découverte, 2017).
5 The biological history of life behind this perspective was pioneered by Lynn Margulis, a collaborator who, with Lovelock, invented the Gaia hypothesis. See her *Symbiotic Planet: A New Look at Evolution* (London: Weidenfeld & Nicolson, 1998).

The New Climate Regime, according to Latour, permits return to the older schema, but as invested with new figures. We now seek "sustainability" against being liberated from the constraints of the cosmos and of civilization, hoping to be able to escape from the end of the world induced by human destructiveness. The end of the world is becoming all too possible, if not inescapable, yet not as the fulfillment of a hope, or as the accomplishment of apocalyptic truth but, instead, as a planetary disaster with heavy human responsibility (96–97). The "end of time" has already arrived for a great part of the species living on earth.

Latour proposes that we stop combatting pagan religions as idolatrous and learn from them, instead, lessons on how to survive (102). The way of "immanence" that they model is about sustainability on a horizontal axis rather than erecting false images of a supposedly transcendent deity or other world. They belong to a regime of truth different from that of monotheistic religions.[6] Both immanence and transcendence are essential registers of figuration for the inexpressible of negative theology, which cannot be contained within either transcendence or immanence to the exclusion of the other.

Discovering and incarnating "the end of time in the time that passes" is the work especially of ritual. Rituals are the key to constructing a common good. Imperative for us is to re-invent for our own time a ritual of the Earth. Latour combines figures of im*man*ence with figures of im*min*ence in order to conjugate the ancestral sanctity of the world with the new urgency necessary to make it not disappear (105). In order to ward off the end of time and the curtailing of our children's future, we must learn immersion and incarnation rather than emancipation. We must learn how to belong and be dependent as a purpose even higher than that of asserting our own autonomy. These are new, but actually age-old, figures that Latour redeploys for reanimating a renewed "apostolic preaching" ("Empêcher la fin du temps, plonger dans les réalités d'en bas, s'immerger et non pas s'émanciper, apprendre à dépendre, voilà le mouvement et l'énergie retrouvée de la prédication apostolique," 107). These renewed figures, moreover, enable preaching the gospel of ecological salvation *ad extra* to those with no background in or inclination to Christianity but with a common stake in the earth and its future.

A question for native communities arises from this critique of liberationist ideology. Is the quest focusing on goals of emancipation and individual sovereignty in line with their ancestral traditions, or is it rather a graft of modern, humanist, anthropocentric culture that betrays the wisdom of their forebears? At least we should consider how to make these revindications in the light of Native American wisdom focused on the

---

6 Latour, *Petite réflexion sur le culte moderne des dieux faitiches* (Paris: La Découverte, 1996) examines this difference in detail.

Eschatology, Incarnation, Kenosis 97

earth as sovereign and as binding us all into mutual dependence rather than releasing us into liberationist autonomy. Native American voices were prophetic in warning against this entire trajectory of the modern world toward liberal emancipation that was such a disaster for their native ways of life.[7] Emancipation and individual sovereignty were not necessary as long as humans lived in intimate connection with other species in the supportive lap of Mother Earth. Maybe they are necessary for subaltern groups in the modern world, with all its forms of subjection and exploitation. But is there not a nuance of difference in the way indigenous peoples might embrace these goals so as not to be simply absorbed into the modern project of emancipation? These are questions as to how native peoples can rebel—or rather guide and lead—along paths other than those of their purported oppressors.

The current crisis requires of all of us a new discipline of self-examination and self-reflection. Ecological eschatology is distinctive in that the end of time is autogenerated. We are ourselves simultaneously the victims and the exterminators (120). Latour foregrounds the *self-reflexive* nature of our current situation and crisis in the New Climate Regime or Predicament as what makes it different from those of the past. This environmental apocalypse, like the modern world itself, is also an apotheosis of self-reflexivity.[8]

Science and religion both need to emancipate themselves from *nature* seen simply as a causal order of laws. They need to become incarnate in the painful birthing of the *flesh* on earth. Latour echoes at this juncture the evangelical language of Saint Paul in Romans 8:25: "For we know that the whole creation groaneth and travaileth in pain together until now." Science and religion, as normative discourses, were both abstract impositions from above. Latour prophetically proclaims the reversal of this orientation in the imperative of our either coming back down to earth or dying. Without taking on prophetic airs himself, he rather ventriloquizes the pope's prophetic voice and message. However, Latour appeals to us not to withdraw and stop development and reverse growth out of respect for nature but rather to *continue* creation by means of ever more intelligent innovation and invention. Ecological eschatology requires us to become *more* artificial rather than less—and more technological than ever. Latour's is a spirituality of the artificial, of the created. This is the creative spirit in which he adopts the prayer to the Lord in Psalm 103:

---

7 T. C. McLuhan, ed., *Pieds nus sur la terre sacrée* (Paris: Denoël, 2021) anthologizes these voices of lucid protest and has become a fundamental reference for general interest in native American culture in France. Original title: *Touch the Earth: A Self-Portrait of Indian Existence* (New York: Outerbridge & Lazaard, 1971).

8 I have developed my own genealogy of modernity as generated by self-reflection in: *Dante's Paradiso and the Theological Origins of Modern Thought: Toward a Speculative Philosophy of Self-Reflection* (New York: Routledge, 2021).

"Thou sendest forth thy spirit, [O Lord], and renewest the face of the earth." We need urgently to apply all the creative capacities of our spirit to the task of renewing the earth and its resources.

There is something absolute and imperative about the theme of the Earth. We have many choices and preferences, but caring for the earth is not an option. It is an absolute condition of our continuing to exist. This is Earth's theological dimension, and it issues in an apocalyptic injunction. It is a negative condition, a condition sine qua non, and as absolute it founds a kind of negative theology. It does not declare a fully articulated positive truth but rather indicates what is essential because without the earth as our ground and support we cannot exist at all. This knowledge is, or should be, enough to unite us in certain directions of effort on behalf of our common salvation.

The positively true and divine remains wide open and impossible to pin down in definitions. Yet the negative realization that everything for us depends on our preserving the earth is the absolute imperative of our lives and thought—their "theological" norm because it transcends us and involves the lives of all the living, at least of all terrestrial beings. Infinite truth and the divine and sacred become possible for us only on the basis of this ground, the ground of the earth. The Earth, as the enabling condition of all life, is a figure for divinity itself. "Earth" is not just a mystifying metaphor but designates imagistically the absolutely real condition of all life. We know this Earth not in the fullness of its own proper essence but only by the negative knowledge that without it we cannot exist. It is something that surpasses our comprehension yet demands all our effort to respect it and act accordingly.

21 Indigenous Salvation as Guide

I resist the idea that we need to reject Western tradition en bloc as transcendentalist and that Indigenous traditions give us the alternative approach to inhabiting the planet that we should have been following all along. However, I wholeheartedly embrace the lessons that can be learned from hearkening to the ancestral wisdom of Indigenous peoples concerning respect and reverence for the Earth. I wish to learn from Indigenous traditions to appreciate more profoundly the forgotten wisdom of the West instead of setting up an invidious opposition, condemning a whole culture and civilization, and pretending to have found *the* salvific alternative.

Indigenous salvation is not to be found somewhere else by abandoning "our" Western culture and history. Salvation or health has to be found dwelling in us and our own cultural ancestry in order to be authentically embodied rather than superficially and perhaps abusively appropriated. It is for this purpose that I wish to renovate and activate the apophatic side of Western speculative tradition.[1] This is one important reason for my taking a traditional great works approach, with emphasis on Western classics, even while searching in the direction of Indigenous salvation, in this quest for a deeper comprehension of the implications of the coronavirus crisis.

The apocalyptic summons that emerged from our survey of world literature in Part I has been taken up and elaborated in some concrete and scientifically precise ways in an apocalyptic register as an eschatology of the earth by Bruno Latour in his later works. Latour's emphasis falls on how new structures of thought are necessary for confronting new and unprecedented challenges to which past forms of thought are no longer adequate. This functionalizing of his thought may well be justified

---

1 I am building here on reflections that I broached in "Unsayability and the Promise of Salvation: An Apophatics of the World to Come," in *Ewiges Leben. Ende oder Umbau einer Erlösungsreligion*, eds. Günter Thomas and Markus Höfner, Religion und Aufklärung series (Tübingen: Mohr Siebeck, 2018), 303–316.

pragmatically, but such a purpose is not the only calling of thought. Thinking is not only for the sake of making new things happen, but also for constructing understanding of where we have come from. This is a crucial part of understanding where we are going. Revisiting the past enables us to transcend the present in projecting the future. This bends linear time into a circular shape such as is more characteristic of indigenous perspectives, with their holistic orientation.

Sean McGrath is consistently critical of forms of "nostalgia" for a sense of wholeness such as the ancient and medieval "cosmos" were supposed to afford. I think, nonetheless, that a form of aspiration to an incompletable wholeness is necessary in order not to betray, by totalization of merely partial perspectives, the quest for truth without arbitrary limits. Constitutive of such thinking is a "contemplative" dimension in the traditional religious vocabulary renewed by McGrath in *Thinking Nature*. I wholeheartedly agree with McGrath in aiming to foster a contemplative attitude in our relation to the real and in not assenting to wholesale rejection of all forms of "transcendence."[2] Such contemplative Western culture is resonantly consonant with Indigenous approaches and rituals for honoring the Earth.

---

2 See McGrath's *Thinking Nature*, particularly its chapters on "Religion Is Not Only the Problem, but Also the Solution," 1–20, and "Contemplative Politics," 138–148, plus 49–50. See, further, Brown and Franke (2016).

22 From "Theology of Hope" to "Theology of the Earth"

Thus, I wish to avoid rejecting Western tradition en bloc as transcendentalist in favor of immanentist approaches such as might be represented by Native American culture. These varying approaches should be used to complement each other by highlighting strengths and weaknesses of one or the other culture. The focus on the Earth in Native American culture can be found echoed also in mainstream Western tradition and notably in Jürgen Moltmann's development of his Scriptural "Theology of Hope" into a kind of "Theology of the Earth." His theology of hope has found a new and timely political application in the ecology movement.

Moltmann's later, earth-oriented theology, too, is elicited from the Bible as a central founding text of Western intellectual and cultural tradition. He crystallized his "theology of hope" in a book of that title published in 1964, but he had elaborated this vision over several decades into an ecologically oriented theology of the Christian doctrine of Creation. His *God in Creation* was first published in 1985 and has been reissued frequently since then.[1] In taking this latter turn, Moltmann works especially from Christoph Blumhardt's theology of the Kingdom of God on Earth. In the expectation and hope of this theology, God's Kingdom comes from the earth and its elements, including water and air, and is an expectation not just *for* the earth but also *of* the Earth as herself an animated subjectivity.

Just as for Latour, so also for Moltmann, we can understand humanity only by thinking it not from itself but rather from the basis of its grounding on the earth ("Um unser Menschsein zu verstehen, müssen wir nicht von uns selbst, sondern von der Erde, ausgehen").[2] Moltmann evokes

---

1 Jürgen Moltmann, Gott in der Schöpfung: Ökologische Schöpfungslehre (Gütersloh: Gütersloher Verlagshaus. 2015 [1985]), trans. *God in Creation: An Ecological Doctrine of Creation* (London: SCM, 1985).
2 Moltmann's essay "Theologie der Hoffnung im 21. Jahrhundert," lays out his transition and his development of his theology of hope into a theology of the Creation and the Earth.

DOI: 10.4324/9781003545835-25

Paul's apocalyptic hope for the freeing of the Creation from its subjection to vanity and perishing:

> For the creation was subjected to vanity, not of its own will, but by reason of him who subjected it, in hope that the creation itself also shall be delivered from the bondage of corruption into the liberty of the glory of the children of God.
>
> (Epistle to the Romans 8:20-21)

The Creation is itself a subject, a person that cries out in agony: "For we know that the whole creation groaneth and travaileth in pain together until now" (Romans 8:22).

This is the birth pang of a new and more just world order that *should* be born and is heard in every cry of the poor of the earth. However, it is still incumbent on us as midwives to bring it into being. This again echoes the theology that Pope Francis magisterially articulated and that so impressed and shook ("ébranlé") Latour and has been transmitted to his followers.[3]

Moltmann can help us to think the pope's analysis through in terms of a theology of the earth building on his own theology of hope. Moltmann reconstructs a biblical theology of the earth in which God, through his promise, bonds himself with the earth directly and not only through humans. The first Creation story in Genesis 1:1-25 establishes the earth as the original source of teeming species, as the motherly womb of life in all its variety. When men resort to killing, first, with Cain's slaying of his brother Abel, God hears a protest coming up from the earth: "I hear the voice of thy brother's blood crying unto me from the ground [or earth]" and pronounces a punishment for the crime "Cursed be the ground [or earth] for your sake" (Genesis 4:10-11). Again, after the Flood, the covenant is made directly with the earth: Yahweh says that the rainbow is set in heaven as a sign of "a covenant between me and the earth" (Genesis 9:13). These passages show that the earth has a direct and privileged relationship with God, one not dependent on or derivative from humans. Of course, humans and their husbandry may still be instrumental in shepherding and protecting God's Creation.

The relation of man and nature in biblical theology cannot be reduced to the commonly cited translations of Genesis 1:28 directing humans to subdue the earth and dominate over other species:

> And God blessed them, and God said unto them, Be fruitful, and multiply, and replenish the earth, and subdue it: and have dominion over the fish of the sea, and over the fowl of the air, and over every living thing that moveth upon the earth.

---

3 Alongside Maniglier as Latour's transmitter, see Frédérique Aït-Touati and Emanuel Coccia, *Le cri de Gaïa, Penser avec Bruno Latour* (Paris: La Découverte, 2021).

Even this statement, read in context, is about caring for and preserving the earth and its creatures rather than exploiting it and destroying them.

There is a biblical humanism that elevates humanity in its freedom over other natural creatures. Yet this means that humanity's free nature, as made in the image of God, gives it a special responsibility for safeguarding and sustaining the order that has been imparted to the Creation by the Creator. This is a different vision from most autochthonous creation myths. Certainly, it can be, and has been, instrumentalized to justify human hegemony. However, it should be read, instead, as a summons to assume a special burden of responsibility for protecting and fostering the Creation.

23 Science, Faith, and Social Belief—Not Strictly Separable

Somewhat similarly to Latour, but from his own philosophical point of view anchored in social theory and political theology, Giorgio Agamben stresses that the dogmatic medical dualism of disease and health presupposes a Gnostic and specifically a Manichean vision.[1] We cannot eradicate disease without eliminating ourselves. Agamben's thinking is nourished by the millenary intellectual, philosophical, and legal tradition of Western culture interpreted in a negative key.[2] Catherine Keller similarly mines rich ore for reflecting on the ecological emergency from such sources in an explicitly negative theological vein.[3] Writing before the Covid-19 crisis, although after Pope Francis, she sounds some of the same alarms and makes the same kind of connections as the pope does between political and environmental injustices. Jürgen Moltmann had already issued a similar warning at a slightly earlier stage of the unfolding environmental disaster in *God in Creation* (1985).

Directly influenced by Agamben, David Cayley offered analysis of the exaggerated reaction called "lockdown" and its hidden motivations along similarly political lines.[4] Cayley brings up an important and revealing issue in pointing out how the governments adopted a rhetoric of the authority of science in order to justify their often excessively repressive measures. Citing his own Canadian authorities in the region of Ontario,

---

1 Giorgio Agamben, "La medicina come religione" and "Distanziamento sociale" online at: https://www.quodlibet.it/giorgio-agamben-distanziamento-sociale. Many of Agamben's writings on this topic are brought together in *A che punto siamo: Epidemia come politica* (Macerata: Quodlibet, 2020), trans. V. Dani as *Where Are We Now? The Epidemic as Politics* (Lanham, MA: Rowman & Littlefield, 2021).
2 I develop a negative theological reading of Agamben's work in William Franke, "Agamben's Logic of the Exception and Its Apophatic Roots and Offshoots," *Concentric: Literary and Cultural Studies* 41/2 (2015): 95-120. Reprised in Franke, *On the Universality of What is Not*, 154-80.
3 Keller, *Political Theology of the Earth: Our Planetary Emergency and the Struggle for a New Public* (New York: Columbia University Press, 2018).
4 https://reviewcanada.ca/magazine/2020/10/the-prognosis/.

DOI: 10.4324/9781003545835-26

he notes how they present science as speaking with one voice. Those who dissent from the prevailing consensus purveyed by the media are discredited as pseudo-scientists.

Scientists of various stripes have produced diverse, sharply clashing and even contradictory views concerning the coronavirus. The gist of the critique of the lockdown strategy was distilled into the Great Barrington Declaration reconceiving the solution through the concept of herd immunity to be developed by exposure of healthy individuals to the virus rather than by lockdown across all sectors of society. Promulgated by three medical specialists in epidemiology from the universities of Oxford, Stanford, and Harvard, the declaration advocated, instead, "Focused Protection" for those vulnerable to severe consequences and death.[5] The policy of having, or even forcing, everyone to avoid all social contacts was seen to be an impediment to developing collective immunity.

A different approach based not on epidemiology but one that analyzes, instead, the social reactions and consequences of the pandemic is put forward by Fareed Zakaria in *Ten Lessons for a Post-Pandemic World*.[6] Zakaria dwells especially on the inequalities that are inevitable but are exacerbated by the Covid-19 crisis and the structural changes to society that it contributes mightily to advancing and accelerating. He places the coronavirus crisis into perspective as aligned with other great shakeups of the nascent millennium, namely, the 2001 terrorist attacks on the World Trade Center and the Pentagon and the 2007–08 global financial crisis provoked by massive debt failure on subprime loans. Each in its way apocalyptic, these events have reconfigured the future and were occasions for radically reconceiving what can be hoped for.

Governments have faced difficult dilemmas in making policy decisions. They have had to pose grave ethical questions—deontology vs. utilitarianism, social solidarity vs. economic sustainability. But they have also taken advantage of the situation in order to consolidate their power and increase disenfranchisement of the common individual, whose basic democratic freedoms have been severely curtailed by using the Covid-19 threat as a pretext for purportedly exceptional measures (for example, interdiction of public assembly in protest movements) that nevertheless encroach on all aspects of normalcy and become increasingly the new normal.

Consequently, a sizable constituency sees the pandemic as primarily a fabrication of the media instrumentalized by elites whose interests are served by concentrating power yet further in the hands of a few. Certainly, large corporations such as Amazon, Google, and Netflix have profited, and paradoxically the stock market reached all-time highs in the midst of unprecedented economic crisis and previously unimaginable creation of

---

5 https://gbdeclaration.org/.
6 Fareed Zakaria in *Ten Lessons for a Post-Pandemic World* (New York: W. W. Norton, 2020).

public debt. Despite repressive measures, persistently dissenting voices and contradictory analyses from medical experts and social analysts have continued to proliferate. Innumerable protests have broken out across countries and continents. The sociology of disease and reactions to it prove to be almost impenetrably complex. Science interacts ambiguously with popular cultural narratives. Priscilla Wald, in *Contagious: Cultures, Carriers, and the Outbreak Narrative* (2008), demonstrates in detail the interaction and contamination between science and cultural narratives about SARS and HIV/AIDS infections. Her work is prescient with regard to the Covid-19 pandemic.

There is certainly an important and urgent wake-up call for us in this pandemic. However, the way it is being treated, as a particular problem objectivized in a specific disease to be eliminated by special technical means, in effect, treats the Covid pandemic as just a passing nuisance to be taken care of and forgotten. That we can defeat this enemy and then return to normal is the message being transmitted together with a number of tacit assumptions that are also subliminally dispatched. We are distracted from the underlying problems that really demand radical change and continuous conversion of lifestyles—conversion of the means and ends of our personal and social existence. We are focused, instead, on getting back to normal—as if that were not already a colossal failure doomed to imminent collapse and too fragile to be sustainable. We prefer the illusion that disease can be overcome by technology without our living more healthily and equitably. We choose to believe that authorities can, and should, find the means to protect us from death and disease.

24 Control and Excess in Dissembling the Unspeakable

Our all-too-human addiction to psychological deceptions and bad faith is an important part of what plagues reveal. Pressed to their limits by plague, our customary systems of dissembling become dysfunctional. Unseemly truths lurch into the daylight. This is already clearly indicated in the classic accounts of plagues describing how they strip away the typical veneers of civilization. Rites of burial of the dead, arguably the oldest and most fundamental of human institutions, are abbreviated and finally abandoned as it becomes impossible to fulfill duties for honoring the dead when the living are barely able to survive themselves. Thucydides already records this specific dysfunction amid general consternation at the collapse of conventional decorum and sacred custom. Boccaccio elaborates grotesquely on it.

Defoe, on the other hand, also notes among the "strange Effects" of plague a strikingly opposite and surprisingly beneficial potential for reconciling humans with one another. Their animosities and prejudices can be suddenly overcome, at least temporarily:

> Here we may observe, and I hope it will not be amiss to take notice of it, that a near view of death would soon reconcile men of good principles one to another ... another plague year would reconcile all these differences, a close conversing with death, or with diseases that threaten death, would scum off the gall from our tempers, remove the animosities among us, and bring us to see with differing eyes than those which we looked on things with before; as the people who had been used to join with the church were reconciled at this time with the admitting the dissenters to preach to them, so the dissenters, who, with an uncommon prejudice, had broken off from the communion of the Church of England, were now content to come to their parish churches, and to conform to the worship which they did not approve of before.
> (174–75)

Among such strange effects, as a flipside of the crisis, literature of the plague, notably Boccaccio's account, reveals, as we have seen, a certain festival aspect with ghastly similarities to the jubilations of the exceptional time of carnival in which laws are suspended and social taboos and interdictions are transgressed. A frenetic activity of life, with all its possible pleasures in excess and without shame or restraint, breaks out under the pressure of plague and produces, by an inverted and perverse logic, a promiscuous mingling of bodies in ways bound to be outlawed under ordinary circumstances. Of course, this extreme behavior was counterpointed by the contrary overreaction of ascetic practices individually and collectively through undifferentiated, draconian lockdowns.

During the Covid-19 crisis, many governments around the world imposed controls on every aspect of life. The state turned into a system of surveillance of citizens, who were no longer allowed to circulate freely. In France, every movement outside of one's home had to be authorized by permissions specifying the times, places, and purposes, of each outing. These permissions were to be downloaded from the internet, printed out, filled in, carried on one's person and shown to law enforcement officials on demand. An incipient model of complete control of life by the State went into action. Such is the state of exception that becomes the norm in Agamben's analyses. Strict regulation of comportments in public and in private unmasks the will for total control on the part of those who govern. This is perhaps simply intrinsic to the nature of any power necessarily conserving and defending itself against all opposition. But it also has a sinister and very disturbing side. It has been chillingly analyzed as the "new totalitarianism" that is led no longer by monstrous dictators but by "dull bureaucrats and technocrats."[1]

Mattias Desmet maintains that totalitarianism is "the logical consequence of mechanistic thinking and the delusional belief in the omnipotence of human rationality" (13). He works from Hannah Arendt's analysis in *The Origins of Totalitarianism* (1951) of isolated atomic individuals, or "atomized subjects," as furnishing the building blocks of totalitarian systems. With his eye on the coronavirus lockdown or "house arrest" rather than on the Nazi and Stalinist regimes analyzed by Arendt, he observes that this insidious technique of "coercive control," too, serves to divide and conquer. He articulates a position more empirically fact-oriented and yet akin to my own, which intensifies and deepens the speculative dimension of this outlook. The book in hand, in effect, responds to Desmet's call for a different "mindset" and fleshes out concretely, based on our forgotten humanities traditions, an alternative view of human identity and relationality within the world, one that abjures thinking that

---

[1] Mattias Desmet, *The Psychology of Totalitarianism* (London: Chelsea Green Publishing, 2022), 7.

further increase in technological sophistication and control alone can solve our problems.

What we discover in the conditions brought on by pandemic is how we are far too complacent in our illusory control over our lives, which nevertheless completely escape us. We have the power to stop ourselves practically from living. Whatever we *can* do becomes practically an obligation, but decisive for our lives is something else entirely. By our reflex to gain control over everything, we have only succeeded in imposing the dictatorship of a technocracy while losing our orientation to the mystery of life and death, which remains beyond us and our control. In hindsight, the closing of schools is now publicly acknowledged, at least in Germany, to have been a huge mistake, not necessary or effective, and to have incurred irretrievable deficits in development among a generation of youths suffering from permanent psychological damage and succumbing often to suicidal impulses.

The traditional Daoist wisdom of China turns on an awareness that willful action aiming to achieve its declared goals bears within it some built-in self-defeating structures and mechanisms. States of overall wellbeing, even ones as simple as a peaceful sleep, are achieved only when they are *not* directly sought out or pursued as such.[2] Of course, that does not prevent us from effectively working to prepare the conditions rendering them possible or even likely. But ultimately what is desired can accrue only involuntarily. Health, too, is ultimately such a gift granted from beyond human control. American Indian approaches honor spiritual powers surpassing the human. We can only acquiesce to them, not command them. This realization can also be reached by a therapeutic analysis of modern society.[3]

The *compulsion to control* that prevents us from recognizing the meaning of pandemic as a call to look beyond our own confidence in technoscientific management is most overwhelmingly manifest in the all-too-human ordering of the concentration camp. Primo Levi is one of a number of authors who invite us to view pandemic disease allegorically through the lens of the Nazi death camps. Social maladies of all sorts have a way of becoming infectious and spreading by dint of the networking nature of social intercourse. Epidemic disease turns up as an obvious and practically ubiquitous symbol for whatever "plagues" human society as such.

---

2 The indispensable source texts are the *Dao-de-jing* and the *Zhuangzi*. Romain Graziani, *L'usage du vide: Essai sur l'intelligence de l'action, de l'Europe à la Chine* (Paris: Gallimard, 2019) interprets and applies their wisdom.

3 This is Hartmut Rosa's endeavor in *Unverfügbarkeit* (Frankfurt a.M.: Suhrkamp, 2018), trans. James Wagner as *The Uncontrollability of the World* (New York: Polity, 2020).

Primo Levi's *If This Is a Man* (*Se questo è un uomo*, 1947) shows how in the death camps the ordinary world of the living is reproduced in intricate and verisimilar detail. The camp, like all modern bureaucratic societies, is run by *funzionari* (officials) and by *prominenti* (individuals of rank, eminences). To the extent that Nazism is analogous to a plague and induces a moral pandemic in humankind (as Camus also insinuates in *The Plague*), we see that one of the results is a hysterical drive to control all aspects of existence, however insignificant or innocuous.

25 Parallel Perspectives and the Novel

A chief purpose of the analyses of pandemics examined here is to place in parallel the medical, social, scientific, cultural, and environmental aspects of the crisis, present and future. It is a crisis of the whole, or rather of neglect of the whole. We cannot defeat the virus as an object or an enemy. We are battling here with and against ourselves as complex systems with life and death both at work within us. This virus, like the classical plagues preceding it, is the revelation of something that we do not want to see or acknowledge, namely, the fact that we are terribly vulnerable to disease and indeed destined to die.

The novelistic treatment of a fictional pandemic by Lawrence Wright in *The End of October* is especially effective in portraying in parallel the different aspects of the life of individuals—Henry Parsons and his wife Jill, his colleague and friend in the World Health Organization, Maria, along with numerous other occasional characters such as his Indonesian taxi driver. The public and the private spheres, and the professional and the personal, are all juxtaposed and turn out to be revealing of one another. It is the whole of our lives in all their aspects that is decisive for determining the fallout from such generalized and uncontainable menaces as pandemics and terrorism. The book opens on a scene placing into tension a Muslim terrorist attack in Rome with the pandemic health threat originating in Indonesia. Both types of menace are apt for captivating exclusive media focus for a moment, and in this regard they are incongruously comparable. Both types of event reveal the nature of our response to such purportedly external threats and also our neglect and blindness to our own unconscious undermining of the basis of our lives and their equilibrium.

The End of October presents a mordant parody of certain personnel working for NGOs, signally, the well-fed Dutch Hans Vattelappesca (a name comically meaning "you go fish"). The serenity and luxury of the World Health Organization's seat in Geneva, Switzerland, are in flagrant contrast with the misery and turmoil of the places in the world that it is supposedly dedicated to serving. This dissonance is augmented by the context of terrorism reaching from the Middle East to Brazil. This contiguous crisis is mentioned as impending and impinging on the other world of cool scientific decision-making concerning medical issues.

State terrorism from Russia, devilishly engineered namely by "Putin," is exposed as laming the US electric power system and cyber network, as well as having unleashed the deadly virus as a biological weapon on the world and precipitating therewith a total breakdown of civil society. The exposure of the endemic hypocrisies of human society and its organizations is appalling, but it is movingly juxtaposed to the heroic struggles of certain individuals to cope with the crisis without renouncing their humanity. This precious dose of invaluable humanity consists not least in an ability to span the tension between diverse domains of activity and responsibility while remaining intact as compassionate, individual persons. This is an exercise that begins with imagining the seemingly impossible.

26 A Semiotic Model of Contagion—Viral Informatics

Priscilla Wald demonstrates how the contagion narrative works at the level of ideas as much as of microbes. She describes how

> the circulation of microbes materializes the transmission of ideas. The interactions that make us sick also constitute us as a community. Disease emergence dramatizes the dilemma that inspires the most basic human narratives: the necessity and danger of human contact.[1]

People want simple solutions. They do not want to face the complexity and contradictoriness of life. Democratic governments naturally seek to cater to these cravings, and the result is unequivocal, yet often contradictory, declarations on all sides that hold all other pronouncements to be false, if not downright imposters. Any kind of common truth, or even basic agreement about facts, becomes difficult or impossible.

In structural ways, the experience of pandemic calls to consciousness universal and inescapable facts that are simply conditions of our existence. Something about the contagion that operates in pandemics is intrinsic to our very nature as signifying beings who live in a symbolic dimension of meaning. Contagion inhabits the nature of the sign. What went viral during the Covid-19 pandemic was, before all, the contradictory information circulating about it and its causes and the cautionary or remedial measures necessary to be deployed against it (masks and vaccinations, chloroquine and quarantine, etc.). Most people experienced the challenges of uncontainable viral infection most immediately in their circuits of information.

Circulation of information offers a dislocating sort of metaphorical displacement of contagious diseases. The general logic of signification in language can be understood on a model of contamination. Such a view is worked out philosophically in subtle detail by Jacques Derrida in *On*

---

[1] Wald, *Contagious: Cultures, Carriers, and the Outbreak Narrative*, 2.

Grammatology (*De la grammatologie*, 1967). As analyzed through Derrida's post-structuralist theory of language, the sign works on a logic of contamination—of the proper by the figural, of the original by the derivative, of the inside by the outside, etc. Once any supposedly alien inflection is given over to signification, it spreads its influence infectiously like a virus, continually mutating and contaminating everything it touches. Through analysis of the workings of language as *(dis)semination* and as an ongoing process of *supplementation*, Derrida shows how communication produces a new kind of corruption with every attempt to reproduce an original meaning or event. We can see in any number of examples how information becomes viral in the age of the worldwide web.

Derrida's radically destabilizing semiotics can be revealing of aspects of our common existence that generally elude us in the ordinary course of our lives and communications but that press in on us with urgency once we are made to arrest normal activity and view the (dys)functioning of our lives as a whole. Just such a self-examination has been provoked and even forced on us by the Covid-19 crisis. The world economy, not to mention the daily activity, the transactions, the comings and goings of ordinary people, were brought to a standstill. No one in the midst of the crisis knew for how long, but the circulation of information and misinformation was inarrestable.

Information, above all, is what goes viral. What has really made the Covid-19 pandemic different from its predecessors is that it took place in our advanced information age when the populations of the world are in unprecedented numbers receiving news, advice, instructions, and regulations that circulate online all around the globe and can reach instantaneously to the ends of the earth. For the first time it has been possible to install a system of control of the movements of whole populations through applications on people's portable telephones. This system, at the same time, enables all manner of false information or "fake news" to spin out of control and allows anonymous, anomalous agents to work their destruction like viruses. Contagion or pandemic is promoted from being a metaphor to being a privileged model for the new and peculiar predicament faced by society in our age of excessive, hypertrophic information and the hyperreality it generates.

27 Hoping against Hope
From Reason to Religion, or Spiritualizing Rationality

HOPE does not have to be stated in a proposition—it does not have to be hope *that* something definable will happen. I take hope more fundamentally as a moral imperative and a religious act of self-surrender to others—to something or someone that is other than ourselves. As such, hope is not distinguishable from faith or love except in its primary orientation to the future. Hope in anything definite is subject to disappointment. But there is also a kind of hope discovered in our touchstone texts that is objectless and absolute: hope against hope (in anything specific). And in spite of hopelessness.

We can find versions of such a perspective on hope in the Bible, especially in its apocalypses, for instance, in Paul's eschatological hope, which abandons everything earthly and objective and imagines another life and world. Such hoping is reflected on in theologies of hope such as Jürgen Moltmann's—centering on the crucified God as giving up all, including life itself, and in the apophatic theology of hope that I have adumbrated here around the problematic of pandemics and the theme of apocalypse. Such hope is native to the realm of religion (or spirituality), I submit, and, like most authentic prayer, is not primarily hope for concrete objects. Abraham receives his son back entire and unharmed, according to Genesis 22, because he relinquished all of his own finite hopes and submitted to God's will that Isaac be sacrificed on Mount Moriah. Abraham is then free to receive in God's measure rather than his own. Kierkegaard's *Fear and Trembling* acutely argues that Abraham's "religious" form of existence reaches beyond the ethical and the aesthetic spheres.[1] John Caputo's life and work apophatically embody such an attitude and approach oriented to the incalculable and unforeseeable, the "impossible," in which alone genuinely religious, prophetic hope can be invested.[2]

---

1 Johannes De Silentio, alias *Søren Kierkegaard, Fear and Trembling: A Dialectical Lyric*, 1843, trans. Walter Lowrie (Princeton: Princeton University Press, 1941).
2 John Caputo, *Hoping against Hope: Confessions of a Postmodern Pilgrim* (Minneapolis: Fortress, 2015), especially 157-67.

Imagining our relation to the All as encompassing us and our belonging to it—and yet as other than all our own means of grasping it—is an existential act to be accomplished in and through hope. By means of hope, we avoid reducing this relation to just one of our own means. This figure of hope can define our relation to God, but other figures are also possible. Non-theistic vocabularies, too, can certainly channel the experience of the sacred through the existential posture of hope as openness to the other—and to the Other as to what (or Who) grants all.

Responding to pandemics tends to aim at fixing things so that the world can go on as before. But apocalypse, by opening to a new and other world, brings with it a wholly different orientation. It can perhaps be crystalized best in a sentiment or emotion without any particular referential content such as is expressed in Julian of Norwich's (1342–1429) famous assurance: "And all shall be well, and all shall be well, and all manner of thing shall be well."[3] Julian herself was stricken ill three times and almost died of plague twice in the river port city of Norwich. The name "Norwich," "north *wic*," from MIddle Saxon *wic* meaning "emporium" or center for crafts and trade, suggests why the town was highly susceptible to all manner of pestilences shipped in from abroad. Here Julian taught, in her revelations or "showings," that "God wishes to cure us of two kinds of sickness; impatience and despair."[4] When the priest administering last rites to her held up a crucifix for her to gaze on in what were supposed to be her last moments, she saw Christ's blood actually flowing from his wounds and received the mystical visions consisting of the sixteen revelations of divine love that are presented in her book.

Julian's is a voice of religious hope resounding out of the dark depths of experience of deadly pandemic disease. She relates to "all" and affirms things altogether in a Christian mystical key that interprets things, however ostensibly negative, as showing a greater and higher power of salvation in the unconditional love of God, which will be all in all in the end. Julian was an anchoress writing her book in an apophatic mystical tradition turned toward the ineffable God. Plague or pandemic becomes the occasion for a showing of the pan-ontological dimension in which all things belong together and in which she sees that they will all be well—regardless of their individual denouements—at a higher, metaphysical level in God's love. Her pronouncement and her vision echoes and answers to God's seeing all that he had created and seeing that it was good (Genesis 1, verses 3, 10, 12, 18, 21, 24, 29).

---

3 Julian of Norwich, *Revelations of Divine Love to Mother Juliana, Anchorite of Norwich*, original 1675 manuscript in British Library. This quintessential statement is quoted and made to resound widely among modern readers by T. S. Eliot in *Little Gidding* (V).

4 The background of this phrase in the context of plagues that nearly killed its author (1342–1417), who is held to be the first English woman to have written a book, is presented by the Reverend Penny Jones online at Julian of Norwich: "all shall be well" (anglicanfocus.org.au). Accessed 3-14-2023.

Source texts such as those evoked in this reflection enable us to place the Covid-19 crisis in a wider human, cosmic, and even ultra-cosmic context concerning the very destiny of human life and existence. They help us to refocus our expectations and hopes and therewith also our endeavors. Hope, I submit, is to be found not in any pragmatic measures that governments can adopt, nor in technical innovations that pharmaceutical companies can invent, but rather in a conversion of life and change of heart. This can be understood as a religious dimension of existence, as in Kant's question "What may we hope for?" ("Was darf ich hoffen") eliciting his philosophy of religion. This inquiry is the sequel to the questions "What can I know?" ("Was kann ich wissen"), which issues in Kant's epistemology, his theory of knowledge, and "What should I do?" ("Was soll ich tun"), which leads to his ethics or moral theory. Kant's critical philosophy answers all these questions self-critically by designating the limits within which human faculties can competently operate. He thereby opens up a space beyond their range for what can only be a matter of faith or hope.

This further dimension of existence to which we are provoked by plague and pandemic is in any case spiritual, and it is wide open to being explored in light of indigenous insights and practices. The original lecture out of which this book has been elaborated was written for an international, interdisciplinary conference attempting to learn from indigenous wisdom placed in parallel with classical traditions concerning values such as vulnerability, gratitude, and survivance, and to plumb how that wisdom enables us to read deeper into these traditional texts as illuminating our contemporary predicament. My hope is that we can face our own dilemmas and vacillations vis-à-vis present and future pandemics a little more wisely with the benefit of this illumination from the millenary human experience and speculative reflection that has accreted and matured around this most exasperating of challenges. The most valid hope that the age-old rites and traditions of humanity enact and vehiculate is rooted in despair about conquering deadly disease once and for all but learning, instead, to live vulnerably in openness to one another and to the radically Other.

It is possible to discern an affinity of this position with classical Christian and Stoic attitudes vis-à-vis plague such as those articulated by Cyprian of Carthage in *De mortalitate*.[5] Indeed, I wish to reconnect with the wisdom of the ages and re-access what may be perennially valid in deep historical tradition. Cyprian wrote in reaction to the plague

---

[5] Cyprian of Carthage, *De mortalitate*, trans. Ernest Wallis as *On the Mortality (or Plague)* (Edinburgh: Eerdmans, 1867). For updated historical information, see Sabine R. Huebner, "The 'Plague of Cyprian': A Revised View of the Origin and Spread of a 3rd-c. CE Pandemic," *Journal of Roman Archaeology* 34 (2021): 151–174. For a critical consideration of Christian and Stoic influences, see J. H. D. Scourfield, "The *De mortalitate* of Cyprian: Consolation and Context," *Vigiliae Christianae* 50 (1996): 12–41.

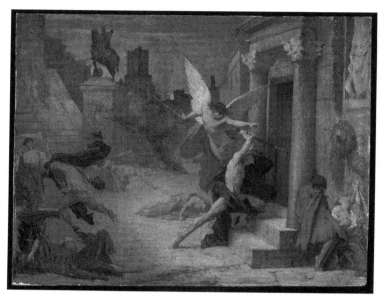

Illustration 27.1 "Roman Plague Allegory," Jules Elie Delauney, 1869.

(known as "Cyprian's plague") that decimated the Roman Empire in the middle of the third century CE and was perhaps an underestimated cause of its downfall.[6] He preaches acceptance of suffering and death. He turns these tribulations into a motive for joy in anticipation of salvation by Christ in his Second Coming and the Apocalypse. Plague has benefits in liberating Christians from this world and in making them hope all the more in the world to come (Illustration 27.1).

This attitude can, of course, come across as sinister to many today. While I think there may be some wisdom in it, I bring it up mostly to stress differences. Such otherworldly promises as Cyprian's "consolatory" homily proffers are transposed by an apophatic or kenotic approach into an eschatologically immanent key emphasizing how attitudes of openness to alterity and acceptance of adversity change our lives and their significance here and now intrinsically, quite apart from whatever may come about in the temporally distant or possibly eternal future. I place the focus, even for Christian ideas of heaven, on how the kind of hope in alterity that I have outlined here has immediate, but also unlimited, life-transforming implications. Such hope issues in engagement with this-worldly imperatives of justice and care.

6 Kyle Harper, *The Fate of Rome: Climate, Disease, and the End of an Empire* (Princeton: Princeton University Press, 2017).

28 Conclusion
Hope-Fail Enactment of Eternity

This book began by observing that the current crisis had the "potentially" salutary effect of revealing us to ourselves. But it is also all too possible to evade this revelation and make of the pandemic just another motive for escape from ourselves and an occasion for denying or ignoring the disturbing fact of our precarious existence. This is especially true as the trauma engendered specifically by the Covid-19 pandemic now begins to recede into the past. Covid has not really changed us and the structure of our society, even though it has accelerated certain tendencies such as the drive to digitalization and to more governmental controls over every sector of human life.[1] New measures such as vaccination passports for travel and perhaps even for going to restaurants, cinemas, and theaters, with attendant obligations of having cellular telephones with surveillance applications making individuals traceable in every aspect of their lives in public and private, have become considerably more palpable looming on the horizon of the future.

What Covid-19 so powerfully and surprisingly revealed is our disturbing willingness and disposition to cede control of all facets of our lives to authorities operating from above. The seriousness of the "pandemic" has been played up by public authorities to the highest pitch in order to catalyze changes in society that already have a strong basis of motivation among governing elites and that have been hovering in the wings, waiting to descend upon social life as upon a prey. Is this not what "lock down," in the phrase we have heard so often, connotes and communicates? On the whole, despite some moaning, we do not want to be responsible for our own health. We prefer to have the government dictate even largely arbitrary—but at least uniform and binding—regulations and so take the responsibility for freeing us of disease and preserving us from death.

---

1 Author Michel Houellebecq ironically issued a reminder that, despite all the upheavals, we will not emerge fundamentally changed from the pandemic but will inevitably seek to return to business as usual. Michel Houellebecq, Coronavirus: pour Michel Houellebecq, le monde d'après "sera le même, en un peu pire" (francetvinfo.fr). Accessed 1-16-2024.

There is arguably some need for general, restrictive legislation. But sought and hoped for as a cure-all, this solution is an illusion and reveals a pathetic need for self-deception more than for free and voluntary individual and collective action in civil society.

Paradoxically, the lack of control that we all experience in pandemics leads to an abdication of control—presumably in the hope that someone else like the government or other higher powers (it used to be the Church) can control what we cannot. Being human is a precarious juggling act of balancing our sphere of personal responsibility and control with our vulnerability to others and our beholdenness to the ultimate mysteries of life and death that we can only honor and acknowledge. Our control is always partial and conditioned by the unknown and unmasterable. Finding our own proper measure in this existential situation can be daunting. The ineffectiveness in the end of all human measures to ward off the plague is a constant motif and a keynote of the literary tradition from Thucydides ("the physicians could do nothing against it," II.47.4) to Boccaccio ("no knowledge or human provision was of any value," 12). It resonates still in Julian of Norwich. The motif of human helplessness in the face of plague continues to crop up among modern writers from Defoe and Manzoni to Camus, Wright, and beyond.

Our reliance on the authority of science often conceals a feint that relieves us of true responsibility for our own health. We prefer to hear that the answers are there and sure and certain if we only consult the qualified, recognized, legitimate authorities. At the same time, a certain repugnance recoiling from such external control and from the dominance of technical measures has also been aroused by recent experience. The latter reaction I hold personally to belong also to the better part of our deeper hope. Yet the tension between alternatives mounts, and the gulf of political misunderstanding deepens and grows more intractable.

At another level, which may seem more abstract and universal, yet is nonetheless real as a reflection in the heart and soul of each person, pandemics in literature are apocalyptic. Pandemics raise questions of the end of the world, or of the viability of human life and society as known hitherto. We are forced to question fundamentally the premises of our existence and the principles of our bonding together and our structuring of society. We are called on to reassess all the hierarchies and inequities that seem inevitably to creep into our relations with one another. All are leveled by disease and death, which are no respecters of persons. Pandemics point up the fragility that is endemic to human life under any circumstances. This makes pandemic a focusing lens for revelation of truth, even of difficult truth, which we usually choose to ignore. It makes pandemic a foyer of hope reaching past the ineliminable threat of disease and beyond the threshold of death that we can hardly fathom, even if we have the courage to try. In this surpassing of ourselves in openness to others and to the Other, I submit, lies our ultimate hope.

This hope directs us beyond our own existence as individuals. Antonin Artaud's reflections on theatre and the plague suggest that experiencing plague can induce a kind of negative attainment of immortality in nonexistence achieved through death.[2] Anaïs Nin reported on Artaud's theatrical enactment of his own death by plague in all its agony in the performing of his essay on "The Theatre and the Plague" as a lecture at the Sorbonne.[3] Her witness supports speaking of Artaud's theatricalization of death by plague as a

> sacrificial gesture. It then becomes a deliberate, voluntary dying that is intended to put death to death, at least virtually, and in so doing, to recover life. At least, such would be the intention that drives 'The Theatre and the Plague.'"[4]

Weber analyzes Artaud's essay as making explicit the "preexisting condition" that the plague serves to highlight, and to such an extent that it "tends almost to eclipse the plague as a self-present event" (141). The preexisting condition is the mortality inherent in each human body, and it takes effect constantly since each person is in the process of dying in every moment of their existence, although this generally passes unremarked. Weber comments that "This eclipse enables Antonin Artaud to portray the plague as an immense, terrible, but also liberating experience—like that of theater" (141). This liberation comes through "the negation of temporal finitude—and inverting it, turning the eternity of nonexistence into a positive quality of the 'self'" (144).

Transcending the self through a theatrical enactment of death can be understood as a realization of eternity. Such an eternity as death (eternal changelessness) can be realized in the experience of confronting the plague, but also in the intensity of the theatrical enactment of death as an apotheosis or apocalypse. According to Nin's recollections concerning Artaud, "He wanted to make people aware that they were dying," but also "to force them into a poetic state."[5]

Picking up on this last suggestion, I would add that Artaud is reenacting here, in a much more demonstrative and pathetic key, and as embodied, the philosophical and poetic drama of Mallarmé's *Igitur*.[6] Igitur struggles with despair, but he turns it into a kind of hope acquired

---

2 Antonin Artaud, "Le théâtre et la peste," in *Le théâtre et son double* (Paris: Gallimard, 1938), 14–36.
3 Anaïs Nin, *The Diary of Anaïs Nin, vol. 1, 1931–1934*, ed. Gunther Stuhlmann (Boston: Mariner Books, 1969).
4 Weber, *Preexisting Conditions*, 143.
5 Anaïs Nin, *The Diary of Anaïs Nin, vol. 1, 1931–1934*, 193.
6 Stéphane Mallarmé, *Oeuvres complètes*, eds. Henri Mondor and G. Jean-Aubry (Paris: Pléiade, 1945).

through relinquishing all hope in anything finite and determinate, a release of his hold on himself as he merges into unity with his ancestors in the tomb. This brings to light an ostensibly somber side of hope in eternity through a tormented and suicidal ceasing to exist that might also be embraced more serenely and sanguinely. The literature we have examined spans the full range of these tonalities. Camus touches deftly on them all.

Camus's novel, which he had originally planned to call *Les séparés* (*The Separated*), situated in the Algerian coastal city of Oran, is strangely concentrated on a European diaspora enclave already enclosed on itself even before the isolation of the plague sets in. There is scarcely any mention of the Arab population. Separation of humans from one another is what the plague figures most profoundly and flushes out into the open. For Samuel Weber, this state of colonial separation is the "preexisting condition" that the plague so poignantly exposes. Denis Guénoun rediscovered this separateness when he revisited his own childhood in Oran in re-reading Camus's novel during the Covid-19 confinement.[7]

Camus's writing traverses the gamut from alarmed panic to serene contemplation. In the concluding Part V of *The Plague*, Camus tellingly states that "One can say, by the way, that from the moment the least hope became possible for the population, the effective reign of the plague was terminated" ("On peut dire d'ailleurs qu'à partir du moment où le plus infime espoir devint possible pour la population, le règne effectif de la peste fut terminé," 245). Hope itself, in this register, is per se the end of the reign of the *pan*dem*ic*. Hope ends panic. In the perspective I have developed here, this is hope not for a "final solution" but hope as an affirmation of life despite its uncontrollable contingency. This is hope not in being able triumphantly to put an end to our vulnerable human condition but rather hope in spite of our helplessness, hope as an unconditional openness to life, including an affirmation of its end.

However, this hope also has an activist and a prescriptive side to it. It frees us for totally committed action in the interest of others. Hope comes in overcoming or suspending the drive to self-preservation and self-aggrandizement at all costs. For this is what breaks down the barriers between us that are the hidden source of our desperation, as well as of our lethal conflicts. Hope that carries us beyond ourselves and our own ambitions, hope for a better world and engagement contributing to a life greater than our own constitute the first steps toward its realization.

---

7 Oran et «La Peste» – Denis Guénoun (denisguenoun.org). Accessed 1-5-2023. https://www.fabula.org/atelier.php?Oran_Camus_la_peste. Accessed 1-5-2023.

29 Coda
Plague and War

Plague comes always, literally or figuratively, entangled with war—another apocalyptic motif. In the Book of Revelation, "There was war in heaven," and Michael and his angels fought against the dragon and his angels and cast them out of heaven (12:7-12). The seven angels carrying vials containing the seven last plagues of the wrath of God pour them out in series and then gather at the place called "Armageddon" (16:17) for cosmic war and the release of the final plagues (Chapters 15:1-16:17). Plague figures imaginatively as a kind of war waged in or by the entire universe.

On a more narrowly localized plain, Homer's plague constitutes a crucial episode in the Trojan War, while Thucydides's narrative of the plague in Athens is intertwined with and sets the scene for his account of the Peloponnesian War. Ovid, too, places plague in the context of war. The war of Athens with Crete is entangled with his account of how a plague was inflicted on the island of Aegina by the goddess Juno in her jealousy against a nymph (Aegina) ravished by her philandering husband, Jove. After the population is decimated, Jove takes pity on their king Aeacus (Achilles's grandfather) and raises the Myrmidons out of a colony of ants to fight for the defense of Athens against Crete mobilized for war by Minos. This passage from Ovid about plague, imaging especially the corruption of human flesh that it causes, is vividly recalled and redeployed by Dante to describe the corrupters of currency, or counterfeiters, in the *Inferno* (XXIX.58-66). Hell is a context of generalized war of all against all.

Defoe mentions repeatedly the trade wars with the Dutch in situating the outbreak of plague in London. And Manzoni traces the Milan plague's origins to Austrian troops and an Italian soldier in the service of the Spanish army as carrier of the plague into the city. He had allegedly bought or stolen infected clothing from Austrian military personnel before visiting his relatives in a village near the eastern gate of the city, where he fell ill and contaminated them. Camus's *The Plague* was written in the aftermath of wartime and as an allegory of war. The consistent association of plague with war cannot be accidental but rather witnesses to some kind of irresistible affinity in their respective imaginaries. Both are discourses of disaster and destruction; both are prone to open into an apocalyptic register of general conflagration and unlimited risk.

Wars and plagues alike are "existential" (as we hear today from political leaders and journalists) and determine what worlds are destroyed and what nations or communities will be given a new lease on life. Lawrence Wright's "Contagion" (the title of his book as translated into Italian and French) plays itself out in the context of an ultimate showdown between Russia and the United States. The "Kongoli" virus itself is produced and spread as part of the arsenal of weapons of mass destruction deployed by these superpowers to destroy one another.

Paul Valery's statement that civilizations learned that they are mortal in the two world wars ("nous autres, les civilizations, nous savons maintenant que nous sommes mortelles"[1]) could apply equally to the pandemics and especially to the Covid-19 pandemic that was globalized in its effects. Both war and plague put at risk our collective survival. We are forced to reconceive our individual being and bodies in relation to the corporate wholes of which they are parts. The boundaries between lives and bodies are reopened in dramatic ways that change our most fundamental perceptions of ourselves.

Although we may wish to resist the analogy between war and pandemic as deployed by governments for political leverage in their efforts to mobilize populations in face of the pandemic, we cannot but recognize its metaphorical power. Moreover, there is an uncannily consistent association of these two extreme forms of disaster throughout literary tradition. Heinrich von Kleist's unfinished tragedy *Robert Guiscard, Duke of the Normans* (*Robert Guiskard: Herzog der Normänner*, 1808) again places plague squarely in the context of war. The plague is decimating the Norman forces besieging Constantinople, just as it did the Greeks before the walls of Troy. The historical, as well as mythic, personage of Ruberto Guiscardo, himself a victim of plague, ends up shining among the blessed warriors in Dante's Heaven of Mars (*Paradiso* XVIII.48). He has been evoked already in the *Inferno* (XXVIII.13-14) in a passage describing the mayhem of historical wars as a comparison for the severed flesh of the schismatics being punished in the ninth *bolgia* or "pouch" of the eighth circle of Hell. This imagery is coordinated with the imagery of plague used for the corruption of the flesh of the counterfeiters—the archetypal "Master Adam" among them—in the ensuing canto, *Inferno* XXIX, and *bolgia* (the tenth).

---

1 Paul Valéry (1871–1945), *La Crise de l'esprit* (1919).

Plague and War   125

Thucydides contemplates the unpredictability of war that makes it strongly analogous to plague. Society and culture endeavor to control time and thereby to render themselves invulnerable and immune to change, but plague, like war, enters the scene to disrupt all such illusory reckonings. Samuel Weber underlines the difference in this respect of the inexplicable striking of plague from the deliberately planned violence of war:

> it is precisely the plague that decisively upsets this project because it is totally incalculable, as incalculable as mortality itself. This is its essential difference from war. In war, the aim is to control mortality by inflicting death upon the enemy and thereby subjugating it.
>
> (64)

This difference is important and helps to elucidate why plague is so peculiarly revealing in the sense of negative theology or unknowability that I have developed here. However, Thucydides constantly dwells on the limits to this ability to predict outcomes in war and on how the longer the war continues the more contingencies enter onto the scene to upset human plans and calculations. The aged Spartan king Archidamus, in his wisdom, points this out in a speech that Thucydides attributes to him (*The Peloponnesian War* I:78).

War and plague alike put human life at dire risk and make us face up to a certain helplessness even in the midst of concerted and, in the end, total effort on our part to protect ourselves and prevail against all insidious and uncontrollable threats. The blurring and breaking down of all distinction between what is deliberately and purposefully accomplished and what happens in spite of our intentions and actions is more nearly what makes plague and war so comparable and almost inseparable. Both catastrophes point up the limit at which human calculations prove vain, even while calling for constant strategic planning and resolute action. This paradoxical pathos places us face to face with the "impossible" or inconceivable (for Camus's humanists).

Franziska Meier points out some inherent limits to first-person narration of plagues.[2] She contrasts plague with war, the latter being a theme that has lent itself better to first-person narration (exemplarily Ernst Jünger's World War I narratives). Certainly, there are some subtle distinctions to be made here, but I think it is mostly a matter of the narrator's distance from or nearness to traumatic events that determines whether

---

2 Franziska Meier, "The Witness: The use of the first-person narrative in the plague descriptions of Thucydides, Giovanni Boccaccio, Daniel Defoe, Alessandro Manzoni, and Albert Camus," *Narrating Pandemics: Transdisciplinary Approaches to Representations of Communicable Disease*, ed. Andrew Gross, Silke Schicketanz and Richard Hoelzl (Toronto: University of Toronto Press, 2025).

first-person narration is necessary or even possible. Either type of event, war or plague, solicits and yet, at the same time, defies first-person narration because as world-shattering experiences they are not rendered adequately by the facts alone and veer into inexpressible registers of awareness that can be conveyed meaningfully only by personal witness. They require irreducibly first-person narration, yet even such direct witness has a strong tendency to issue in silence. Dante, at the height of the *Paradiso*, invoking the ineffability of his final vision of God, performs this predicament paradigmatically in the last canto, 33, as an elaborate liturgy on its own impossibility.[3] Thus ends the infernal war and purgatorial purging of the plague of sin.

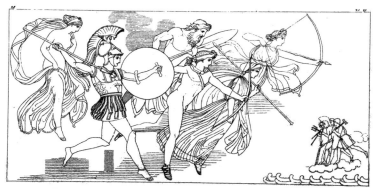

Illustration 29.1 "Gods Descending to Battle," John Flaxman's Iliad, 1795.

---

3 See my "The End of Imagination (*Paradiso* 33)," *Project* Paradiso: *A Gateway to Dante's Heaven*, eds. Filippo Gianferrari and Ronald Herzman (New York: Routledge, forthcoming).

30 Appendix
Abstracts of Selected Plague Narratives in Literature, Classical to Modern

The biblical Book of **Exodus** (7:14–10:20) describes ten plagues wrought by God and brought down calamitously on Pharaoh and his people in Egypt until he stops refusing to let the enslaved people of Israel go. The term "plague" is used here generically, as is often the case, for all sorts of natural disasters afflicting human and animal life and menacing both with precipitous death in masses. The ten plagues include (1) the pollution of the Nile with blood; (2) the covering of the land of Egypt with frogs; (3) dust turned to noisome gnats (or possibly lice); (4) swarms of flies (or possibly wild animals); (5) pestilence upon livestock; (6) festering boils on the skin of humans and animals; (7) fire and hail raining down from heaven; (8) locusts devouring everything in the land; (9) darkness over the land of Egypt for three days; (10) and finally the death of all firstborn sons. These plagues are "signs and wonders" (Exodus 7:3-4) demonstrating to the Egyptians that Israel's Yahweh is truly God. That such "plagues" are inflicted by God on humans for their sins is archetypal and becomes constitutive of the very concept of plague, at least in its more deeply embedded, unconscious significance.

The "plague" at the outset of **Homer**'s *Iliad*, Book 1 is caused by the god Apollo, "the archer who kills from afar." He slays the Greeks because his priest, Chrises, has been refused in a suit to ransom his daughter, Criseide. She is being held captive as his concubine by the Greek leader and general, Agamemnon. The soothsayer, Calchas, reveals this as the cause of the pestilence. Agamemnon decides to take the war-booty concubine Briseis away from Achilles to replace the one that he is constrained to give up in order to satisfy the god and end the pestilence. In this manner, the Western epic tradition begins precisely with a plague caused by a god punishing humans. This original source text also connects plague with war and thereby inaugurates another, equally long history and tradition. Devastating destruction by human hands with weapons bleeds into and becomes one with even greater, unsparing destruction of human lives by disease. The mystery of death and destruction as having some kind of enigmatic necessity (*Ananke*, ἀνάγκη) to which humans can only submit dances over the spectacle of human perishing like a divine destroyer (Shiva), even while humans make reparations and attempt to placate the gods.

Sophocles's *Oedipus Rex*, circa 429–25 BCE, represents the plague in Athens as caused by Oedipus's unconscious crimes of patricide and incest. This classic work highlights an apparently unavoidable unknowing of oneself yet at the same time unflinchingly affirms the fatal consequences of this ignorance. The integration of an ethical cause of plague, a specific human transgression, into its human and social tragedy contains an element of rationalizing explanation. King Oedipus himself, in his determination to bring to the light of day the cause of the mysterious miasma, epitomizes the hero of uncompromising rationality. But this does not prevent the choruses from amplifying the plague's metaphysical significances as a kind of religious pollution, lending it a mythological dimension that looms large in depictions throughout later literature. **Seneca**'s *Oedipus* (lines 52–201), in the first century CE, plays up, with characteristic pathos, the cosmic and apocalyptic resonances of pestilence in this archetypal drama.

Thucydides's account of the plague in Athens in 430–426 BCE at the beginning of the Peloponnesian war stands unrivalled as a classic model of historiography. The Spartan invasion causes villagers living in the country around Athens to take refuge in the city, and this concentrates a contagion perhaps of typhoid fever, making the epidemic the more virulent. This "plague" is described in a detached tone and in exacting detail by Thucydides in his *History of the Peloponnesian War* (II.47–54). He considers the plague to be a chief cause of Athens's defeat in the war against Sparta (III.87), although he refrains from speculating about the plague's own causes (περὶ αὐτοῦ ... τὰς αἰτίας), leaving that to others (II.48.3). He furnishes clinically objective analysis of medical and epidemiological aspects (drawing on the Hippocratic school of medicine), as well as of the sociological consequences of the breakdown of law and order in the face of immanent and arbitrary death.[1] The disturbing description of a general collapse of morals in the wake of the plague calls into question and implicitly undermines Pericles's ringing celebration of the noble virtues of the Athenians in his famous funeral oration. The oration is reported in the immediately preceding chapters of Thucydides's history (II.34–46) that form a diptych with his plague narrative. Thucydides's plague description becomes the template for the more demonstratively poetic, emotionally colored, and psychologically slanted reflections of Lucretius. The latter's more pathetic treatment was widely disseminated and influential throughout Latin and Western tradition.

---

1 Thomas E. Morgan, "Plague or Poetry? Thucydides on the Epidemic at Athens," *Transactions of the American Philological Association (1974-2014)* 124 (1994): 197–209.

Lucretius, *De rerum natura* VI.1090–1286, treats the plague at Athens, dramatizing and psychologizing the account given by Thucydides. Nevertheless, Lucretius, as a natural philosopher, discerns natural causes for the plague, which he attributes to germs contaminating air and water. Whereas Thucydides had said that he was incapable of explaining the causes (*aitia*) and left that to other writers (II.48.3), Lucretius concentrates on explaining the material causes and provenance ("ratio ... aut unde") of plague (1090–1137). He ascribes it to infection of the air by malignant atoms. His account is considerably more pathetic than Thucydides's clinical descriptions and is also more desacralizing, adding a note of scorn to the observation of the futility and impotence of religion. He dwells on the sacrileges committed by the dying and by those attending to them. Yet Lucretius's ending his epic with this triumph of death through the devastation of the plague highlights limits to human powers that even his Epicurean optimism cannot avoid admitting and acknowledging. Naturalist critic of religion that he is, Lucretius nonetheless brings on the plague, giving it the last word, as his work's final disclosure and as a sort of apocalypse. The inscrutable mystery of nature and its tragic perverseness remains as an inexpungible truth overshadowing and giving the lie to the rational enlightenment proffered by his naturalistic philosophy. It is a jarringly tragic conclusion to a profoundly reflective poem based on, but in the end contradicting, Epicurus's optimistic philosophy of happiness.

Virgil, *Georgics* III.478–566 (finale), follows much in Lucretius's plague narrative, projecting it onto the plague of Noricum (in the East Austrian Alps) and amplifying it into a kind of cosmic pain. The plague comes down upon creatures as an act from heaven ("morbo caeli"). Virgil describes chiefly an animal plague and does so in elegant, exquisitely wrought language. This displacement dramatizes but also distances. We are able to contemplate loss of livestock somewhat more objectively and dispassionately when our own skin seems not to be directly at risk, and yet Virgil anthropomorphically projects human emotions onto his scenes of animal suffering. He introduces a highly subjective style in imagining the pathetic demise of each species of animals, both domestic and wild. Virgil confirms the move from observation and exact description to an attitude of literary elaboration and contemplation of the plague in its cosmic significance that is already intimated in Lucretius. This is the heritage profoundly at work already also in Greek tragedy (with *Oedipus Rex*). Virgil effects a transposition into a rhetorical register without regard for clinical credibility. The latter had remained primary still in Lucretius, but Virgil makes the elegance of the writing more important than accuracy and verisimilitude in the description. "This is legend, pathos, writing for effect.

It is not science, or history."[2] A significant consequence is that plague is approached not just as an objective event in the external world but as a subject of poetic revery and artificial literary elaboration. It stimulates a heightened reflexivity in meditative reflection on the universal condition of the cosmos.

Ovid, *Metamorphoses*, VII.523–613, also works from Lucretius, as well as from Virgil, in creating an imaginative apotheosis of the plague of Aegina caused by the goddess Juno's anger. The vengeance of Juno for Jupiter's infidelity with the nymph Aegina brings pestilence down on this small island south of Athens. Such an explanation might give a sense of knowing, and therewith of being able to master, the causes. Such is certainly at least one traditional function of myth. Indeed, Ovid notes that medical science was employed to combat the plague only as long as its causes were unknown (VII.525–27). Once the plague is known to have been sent by the gods, there is no longer any hope, certainly not in medicine. Ovid then describes the hopelessness engendered by the plague and its sure death, against which nothing was of any use—but also the libertarian indulgence that this induces by removing all sense of shame ("positoque pudore," 567):

> ... utque salutis
> Spes abiit finemque vident in funere morbi,
> Indulgent animis et nulla, quid utile, cura est;
> Vtile enim nihil est
>
> (VII.564–67)
>
> ... and as the hope of salvation
> vanishes and they see the end of the sickness in death,
> they indulge their instincts and give no heed to anything
> that is useful; for nothing is useful.

Nevertheless, in spite of all, language lends its unique resources for the conceiving of a new beginning after the decimation of King Aeacus's people. Myrmidons (from the Greek μύρμηξ-*myrmex* for "ant") arise from ants to repopulate the island. This demonstrates, or at least indirectly suggests, how language for the poet serves to create a new world and to symbolize the possibility of the world being remade from its ashes and rising up again like the phoenix.

In *Inferno* XXIX.58–66, **Dante** evokes the plague of Aegina described by Ovid as an image of devastating and pervasive sickness. Their diseased

---

[2] David West, "Two Plagues: Virgil, *Georgics* 3.478-566 and Lucretius 6.1090-1286," *Creative Imitation and Latin Literature*, ed. David West and Tony Woodman (Cambridge: Cambridge University Press, 2010), 72.

flesh makes outwardly manifest the sin of the counterfeiters in corrupting precious metals. The sinners' skin is corrupted as a metaphorical display of the alloying of precious metal that was the transgression against the health of the commonwealth committed by the counterfeiters. They had adulterated its currency and therewith the lifeblood circulating in its veins. In the present context, it is surely worth recalling that Dante (1265–1321) is also widely appreciated as the "prophet of hope" ("profeta di speranza"), to repeat Pope Francis's tribute on the occasion of the 700th centenary of the poet's death.[3] This appreciation moves beyond Dante's more well-known fame as the poet of hellfire and damnation. Dante's hell graphically embodies the notion of human sin as tantamount to a pervasive sickness or pandemic, even as a congenital disease (following an Augustinian conception), since he accepts the Church's doctrine that baptism is necessary for redemption and healing from Original Sin. Nevertheless, Dante's emphasis falls foremost on the free choice of individual sinners or saints. This is what is made manifest by the punishments and rewards eternalized in the afterlife Dante depicts.[4] Here, too, Dante does not diverge from his predecessor, Augustine. Where there is free will, there is hope ("mentre che speranza ha fior del verde," *Purgatorio* III.135). And this hope is realized in significant exceptions to the law of no salvation outside the Church: Trojan Riphaeus and the Roman Emperor Trajan, known to the world as pagans, are astonishingly saved and beatified in *Paradiso* XX. The concluding 33 verses of *Paradiso* XIX detailing the egregious misdeeds of Europe's Christian princes form, in contrast, an acrostic spelling the word for plague "LUE" (Latin: *luēs*) by repeating each of these letters three times at the head of three successive tercets each. The injustice of hypocritically Christian leaders is thus inscribed as plague iconically into Dante's text.

Boccaccio, *Decameron* (1353), takes the Black Death in Florence in 1348 as the frame for the fiction. In contrast with this frame, the hilarious, satirical, salacious, and irreverent stories of the novellas offer much that is light and frivolous farce. The reading given here concentrates almost exclusively on the frame story, yet its juxtaposition to the one hundred entertaining novellas cannot but reflect on and accentuate its gruesome content. A contrapuntal pathos rebounds to the stories from their enframement by the plague, and the plague, too, is seen in a very different light once it is distanced into the background and becomes an invisible backdrop for

---

3 Pope Francesco, *Candor lucis aeternae*. Lettera apostolica in occasione del VII centenario della morte di Dante Alighieri (Milan: Paoline, 2021), 29–32.

4 In *The Revelation of Imagination: From Homer and the Bible through Virgil and Augustine to Dante* (Evanston: Northwestern University Press, 2015), chapter 5: Dante's Poetics of Revelation, 307–384, I elucidate how the punishments are simply the manifest expression of the sins as they are presently committed by the souls even as Dante encounters them in the afterlife.

stories exploring the comic and dramatic aspects of human experience in all its vanity and glory. All this might ordinarily be brought to naught by as serious and sobering a subject as the plague, of which Boccaccio delivers a masterful, psychologically and sociologically penetrating analysis.

Defoe, *A Journal of the Plague Year* (1722), offers a fictionalized chronicle looking back on the plague in London in 1635. Although Defoe also published a treatise called *Due Preparations for the Plague, as well as for Soul as Body* (1722) shortly before the *Journal*, he deemed the fictional account to be the more important and effective means to reach people and alert them.[5] Having witnessed the considerable success of his first-person novels *Robinson Caruso* (1619) and *Moll Flanders* (1622), he had discovered the very great potential of fiction to convert hearts and influence behavior.

The narrator is identified in the end simply by the initials "H. F." of Defoe's uncle, Henry Defoe, who, unlike Daniel, would have been of an age to experience the 1635 plague in full cognizance and serve the author as source of information. While representing himself as a pious believer in God's goodness and providence, the narrator is confronted with the much more skeptical and even blasphemous views of free thinkers in the supposedly enlightened society surrounding him. This creates a certain dialectic between scientifically enlightened versus religious understandings of the plague, although the narrator is set in his convictions and not inclined to self-questioning. The conflict is nonetheless central to modern culture struggling with the recrudescence of infectious disease as a withering comeuppance that gives the lie to the modern myth of progress. Defoe's reflection sticks very much to facts and to anecdotes from daily life and yet is on its way to the excruciating and tormented treatment given to this question of the metaphysical meaning of plague and pestilence by Manzoni, where rationalism and fideism vie with one another, neither being quite able to overcome the other.

Manzoni's *The Betrothed* (1844) is an historical novel pivoting on the upheavals wrought by plague in Milan in the 1630 pandemic. Manzoni plays human responsibilities off against narratives of divine punishment and irrational astrological explanations, but the excessive nature of the pandemic defies explanation altogether and opens another dimension of awareness and relation to what is beyond human control. A Christian providential view of history emerges from the novel as its overarching message incarnate in heroic characters, particularly in prelates such as brother Cristoforo and Federigo Borromeo (1564–1631), the famous Milanese cardinal. Both sacrifice themselves for love of others and incarnate the grace of forgiveness or pardon ("il perdono") as a truly redemptive and salvific power. The calculations of reason can offer little to compare in majesty

---

5 Daniel Defoe, *A Journal of the Plague Year*, ed. Paula R. Backscheider (New York: Norton, 1992), ix.

and dignity with this colossal human, not to say divine, passion of charity projected onto an epic scale in the ultimately Romantic vision of the novel.

Edgar Allen **Poe**'s tale "The Mask of the Red Death" (1842) defeats the idea that a retreat to the country can put a select society out of range of the plague. This allegorical tale contemplates human defenselessness in the face of death from infectious disease. It offers another briefer testimony of how the imagination seizes the apocalyptic implications of plague and human helplessness and explores them in a key of Gothic horror.

Antonin **Artaud**, "Le théâtre et la peste," in *Le théâtre et son double* (1938), approaches the plague in Marseille in 1720 through the lens of a dream vision. Artaud emphasizes the analogy between plague and theatre as parallel and "beneficent" means of stripping away masks and forcing us to see ourselves as we are. Like theatre, plague reveals to us our hypocrisy and baseness, our spinelessness and mendacity ("l'action du théâtre comme celle de la peste, est bienfaisante, car poussant les hommes à se voir tels qu'ils sont, elle fait tomber le masque, elle découvre le mensonge, la veulerie, la bassesse, la tartuferie," 36). Plague and theatre are comparable as both "revelations" of "latent cruelty" (34), and they perform alike in serving important cathartic purposes in society.

Albert **Camus**, *La peste* (1947), stages plague as an allegory of the occupation of France by the Nazis and the dilemmas of attempting to resist it. Although the virtues of solidarity and patient scientific analysis are modeled by the physician protagonist, Dr. Rieux, his resistance alone does not emerge as sufficient to clearly win the day. Humanist values show up not triumphantly and heroically so much as being necessary but somewhat pious wishes ("voeux pieux") that can never definitively root out evil, which comes and goes, and abides its time in ambush. At the very end of the book, with the plague's vanishing,

> Rieux ... knew what the crowd in its joy ignored, which can be read in books, that the germ of the plague does not die nor ever disappear, that it remains for decades dormant in furniture and linen, that it patiently waits in bedrooms and cellars and trunks, in handkerchiefs and piles of papers, and that the day perhaps would return when, for the misfortune and education of humans, plague would reawaken its rats and send them to die in a happy city.

> Rieux ... savait ce que cette foule en joie ignorait, qu'on peut lire dans les livres, que le bacille de la peste ne meurt ni ne disparaît jamais, qu'il peut rester pendant des dizaines d'années endormi dans les meubles et le linge, qu'il attend patiemment dans les chambres, les caves, les malles, les mouchoirs et les paperasses, et que, peut-être, le jour viendrait où, pour le malheur et l'enseignement des hommes, la peste réveillerait ses rats et les enverrait mourir dans une cité heureuse.

> (279)

The plague remains always with us because it remains within us, even though external materials and objects are ticked off as the circumstances in which it lingers, biding its time. This recognition belongs to the human self-reflection that is so necessary, beyond whatever medical and technological advances, in Camus's vision.

Lawrence **Wright**'s novel *The End of October* (2020) brings the contemporary dismay and panic over war and terrorism together with infectious disease turning into pandemic in a dramatically apocalyptic perspective of Armageddon. Putin's Russia takes advantage of biological weaponry to inflict the "Kongoli" virus on the entire world, although Henry Parsons of the CDC (Centers for Disease Control and Prevention) working for the United States also bears a certain sense of scientific responsibility for this catastrophe. The novel orchestrates diverse aspects and registers of human life across the entire globe. This makes it a powerful revealer of the capaciousness of the novel as a genre peculiarly fit to treat as gigantic a subject as pandemic with the breadth and expansiveness that it demands. Written and marketed as a thriller, the novel belongs to a genre of popular culture, but this should not be taken as a reason to sell short the imaginative breadth and prophetic insight that has gone into its making. A revolution in recent academic study has reversed the supposed inferiority of popular culture to "high culture." Popular genres have means of working powerfully on the emotions, and this is highly relevant to inducing a state of visionary insight.

Attributing a certain kind of prophetic office and efficacy to Wright's thriller may not be as far-fetched as it at first seems if we understand the novel in a negative theological register. Slavoj Žižek has suggested that horror films may be the true and authentic negative theology of our time: "I think horror films are the negative theology of today. I don't think we can understand the logic of negative theology without appreciating good horror movies."[6] He says this because horror films introduce an element of the "alien" that organizes itself and operates quite beyond our ability to control or even to fathom it.[7] We are forced to face our limitations and impotence. Žižek has provocatively reconceived Christian theology around the idea of its fruitful failure.[8] However, theology's inevitable failure, based on human incapacity to conceive of transcendent divinity, is foundational for the discipline and genre understood from the perspective of classical apophatic or negative theology. It is precisely in taking consciously to heart our human failing that we can be broken open and made receptive to the divine beyond our own capacities. In this hope-fail sense, we are fulfilled/failed.

6 Slavoj Žižek, "A Meditation on Michelangelo's Christ on the Cross," in Milbank and Žižek, *Paul's New Moment: Continental Philosophy and the Future of Christian Theology*, ed. Creston Davis (Grand Rapids: Brazos Press, 2010), 169–182. Citation, 80.
7 Aaron Daniels organizes the burgeoning literature around aliens in *A Phenomenology of the Alien: Encounters with the Weird and Inscrutable Other*, ed. Aaron Daniels (New York: Routledge, 2025), forward by William Franke.
8 See Marika Rose, *A Theology of Failure: Žižek Against Christian Innocence* (New York: Fordham University Press, 2019).

Bibliography

Aït-Touati, Frédérique and Emanuel Coccia (2021) *Le cri de Gaïa, Penser avec Bruno Latour*. Paris: La Découverte.

Agamben, Giorgio (2020) *A che punto siamo: Epidemia come politica*. Macerata: Quodlibet. Trans. V. Dani as *Where Are We Now? The Epidemic as Politics*. Lanham, MA: Rowman & Littlefield, 2021.

Artaud, Antonin (1938) "Le théâtre et la peste." In *Le théâtre et son double*. Paris: Gallimard. 14–36.

Augustine, Saint (c. 400) *Confessiones*. Trans. as *Confessions*. Ed. James J. O'Donnell. *Confessions*. 3 vols. Oxford: Clarendon Press, 1992.

Augustine, Saint (c. 418) *De gratia Christi et de peccato originali*. CSEL (Corpus Scriptorum Ecclesiasticorum Latinorum) 42, 202 [23–25]. Patrologiae cursus Completus: Series Latina. Ed. J. P. Minge. Paris: Migne, 1844–1864. Trans. as On the Grace of Christ and on Original Sin, 2024.

Augustine, Saint (c. 426) *De civitate Dei*. Ed. David Knowles. Trans. Henry Betterson. New York: Penguin, 1972.

Barthes, Roland (1955) "La *Peste*: Annales d'une épidémique ou roman de solitude?" *Club*, February: 6, *Œuvres complètes*, 540–541.

Bellah, Robert N. and Hans Joas, Eds. (2012) *The Axial Age and its Consequences*. Cambridge, MA: The Belknap Press of Harvard University Press.

Bible. The King James Version of the Holy Bible (Authorized Version). http://www.davince.com/bible

Bloch, Ernst (1918/1923) *Geist der Utopie*. Munich and Leipzig: Duncker & Humblot. Trans. Anthony A. Nasser as *The Spirit of Utopia*. Stanford: Stanford University Press, 2000.

Bloch, Ernst (1954-59) *Das Prinzip Hoffnung*. Berlin, Aufbau. 3 vols. Trans. Neville Plaice, Stephen Plaice, and Paul Knight as *The Principle of Hope*. Boston: MIT Press, 1995.

Boccaccio, Giovanni (1985) *Decamerone*. Ed. Vittorio Branca. Milan: Mondadori.

Boccaccio, Giovanni (2016) *Decameron*. Ed. Wayne A. Rebhorn. New York: Norton.

Brown, Nahum and William Franke, Eds. (2016) *Transcendence, Immanence, and Intercultural Philosophy*. London: Palgrave Macmillan.

Butler, Judith (2022) *What World is This? A Pandemic Phenomenology*. New York: Columbia University Press.

Camus, Albert (1947) *La peste*. Paris: Gallimard.

Camus, Albert (1964) *Carnets: Janvier 1942-Mars 1951*. vol. 2. Paris: Gallimard. Trans. Justin O'Brien as *Notebooks: 1942-1951*. New York: Knopf, 1966.

Caputo, John (2015) *Hoping against Hope: Confessions of a Postmodern Pilgrim*. Minneapolis: Fortress

Ceruti, Mauro and Francesco Bellusci (2023) *Umanizzare la modernità: Un modo nuovo di pensare il futuro*. Milan: Cortina.

Civitarese, Giuseppe, Walter Minella, Giannino Piana, Giorgio Sandrini, Eds. (2020) *L'invasione della vita: Decisioni difficili nell'epoca della pandemia*. Milan: Mimesis.

Cone, James H. (1969) *Black Theology and Black Power*. New York: Harper&Row.

Cyprian of Carthage (1867) *De mortalitate*. Trans. Ernest Wallis as *On the Mortality (or Plague)* Edinburgh: Eerdmans.

Daniels, Aaron, Ed. (2025) *A Phenomenology of the Alien: Encounters with the Weird and Inscrutable Other*. Psychology & the Other series. Ed. David Goodman. New York: Routledge.

Danowski, Déborah and Eduardo Viveirso de Castro, Eds. (2017) *The Ends of the World*. Cambridge: Polity Press.

Das, Saitya Brata (2023) *Political Theology of Life*. Eugene, Oregon. Pickwick Publications.

Defoe, Daniel (1992) *A Journal of the Plague Year*. Ed. Paula R. Backscheider. New York: Norton.

Defoe, Daniel (1896 [1722]) *Journal of the Plague Year*. Ed. George Rice Carpenter. New York: Longmans, Green, and Co. Available online at Internet Archive and Gutenberg as: "A Journal of the Plague Year, Being Observations or Memorials, Of the most Remarkable Occurrences, As well Publick as Private, which happened in *London*, During the last Great Visitation in 1665, Written by a Citizen who continued all the while in London. Never made public before." Accessed from www.gutenberg.com on 3/6/2023.

Deloria, Vine Jr. (1973) *God is Red: A Native View of Religion*. New York: Putnam.

Delumeau, Jean (1978) *La peur en Occident XIVe-XVIIIe siècle*. Paris: Fayard.

Derrida, Jacques (1989) "No apocalypse, not now: à toute vitesse, sept missives, sept missiles," in *Les Cahiers du GRIF*, 41–42, L'imaginaire du nucléaire. Trans. Catherine Porter and Philip Lewis as "No Apocalypse, Not Now (Full Speed Ahead, Seven Missiles, Seven Missives)". *Diacritics* 14/2, Nuclear Criticism (1984): 20–31.

Derrida, Jacques (1993) *Sauf le nom*. Paris: Galilée.

Derrida, Jacques (2001) "Non pas l'utopie, l'im-possible." In *Papier Machine*. Paris: Galilée.

Desmet, Mattias (2022) *The Psychology of Totalitarianism*. London: Chelsea Green Publishing.

Bibliography 137

Dupuy, Jean-Pierre (2021) *La catastrophe ou la vie: Pensées par temps de pandémie*. Paris: Seuil.

Eagleton, Terry (2015) *Hope without Optimism*. Charlottesville: University of Virginia Press.

Ferry, Luc (2016) *La révolution transhumaniste: Comment la technomédecine et l'uberisation du monde vont bouleverser nos vies*. Paris: Plon.

Francis, Pope (2015) Encyclical *Laudato si'* "Praised be" ("On the Care of Our Common Home"). Libreria Editrice Vaticana. Laudato si' (24 maggio 2015) | Francesco (vatican.va). Accessed 3-13-2023. English print edition: *Encyclical on Climate Change and Inequality: On Care for Our Common Home*. Brooklyn: Melville, 2015.

Francis, Pope (2021) *Candor lucis aeternae*. Lettera apostolica in occasione del VII centenario della morte di Dante Alighieri. Milan: Paoline.

Franke, William (1993) "Poetics and Apocalypse in Manzoni's Interpretation of History." *Esperienze letterarie* XVIII - n. 4: 17–38.

Franke, William, Ed. (2007) *On What Cannot Be Said: Apophatic Discourses in Philosophy, Religion, Literature, and the Arts*. Notre Dame: University of Notre Dame Press. 2 vols.

Franke, William (2015) *The Revelation of Imagination: From Homer and the Bible through Virgil and Augustine to Dante*. Evanston: Northwestern University Press.

Franke, William (2018) "Unsayability and the Promise of Salvation: An Apophatics of the World to Come." *Ewiges Leben. Ende oder Umbau einer Erlösungsreligion*. Eds. Günter Thomas and Markus Höfner, Religion und Aufklärung series. Tübingen: Mohr Siebeck.

Franke, William, Ed. (2020) *On the Universality of What is Not: The Apophatic Turn in Critical Thinking*. Notre Dame: University of Notre Dame Press.

Franke, William (2021a) *Dante's* Paradiso *and the Theological Origins of Modern Thought: Toward a Speculative Philosophy of Self-Reflection*. New York: Routledge.

Franke, William (2021b) "Amphiboles of the Postmodern: Hyper-Secularity or the Return of the Religious?" *Sacred and the Everyday: Comparative Approaches to Literature, Religious and Sacred*. Ed. Stephen Morgan. Macau: University of Saint Joseph Academic Press. 9–33.

Franke, William (2023) "Not War, Nor Peace. Are War and Peace Mutually Exclusive Alternatives?" *War: Thinking the Unthinkable*. Eds. Cindy Zeiher and Mike Grimshaw. Special Issue of *Continental Thought and Theory: A Journal of Intellectual Freedom* 4/1: 25–35.

Franke, William (2025) "The End of Imagination (*Paradiso* 33)," *Project Paradiso: A Gateway to Dante's Heaven*, Eds. Filippo Gianferrari and Ronald Herzman, New York: Routledge.

Frege, Gottlob (1892) "Über Sinn und Bedeutung." *Zeitschrift für Philosophie und philosophische Kritik* 100: 25–50. Trans. M. Black as "Sense and Reference." *The Philosophical Review* 57 (1948): 207–23.

Girard, René (1982) *Le bouc émissaire*. Paris: Grasset. Trans. Yvonne Freccero as *The Scapegoat*. Baltimore: Johns Hopkins University Press, 1986.

Gomel, Elana (2000) "The Plague of Utopias: Pestilence and the Apocalyptic Body." *Twentieth Century Literature* 46/4: 405–433.

Graziani, Romain (2019) *L'usage du vide: Essai sur l'intelligence de l'action, de l'Europe à la Chine*. Paris: Gallimard.

Guttiérez, Gustavo (1971) *Teología de la liberación. Perspectivas*. Lima: CEP. Trans. Caridad Inda and John Eagleson as *A Theology of Liberation: History, Politics, and Salvation*. Maryknoll: Orbis, 1988; 1st ed., Maryknoll: Orbis, 1973.

Hadot, Pierre (2004) *Le voile d'Isis. Essaie sur l'histoire de l'idée de nature*. Paris: Gallimard. Trans. Michael Chase. *The Veil of Issis: An Essay on the History of the Idea of Nature*. Cambridge: The Belknap Press, 2006.

Harper, Kyle (2017) *The Fate of Rome: Climate, Disease, and the End of an Empire*. Princeton: Princeton University Press.

Heidegger, Martin (1949) *Über den Humanismus*. Frankfurt am Main: Klostermann. Translated as "Letter on Humanism." In Martin Heidegger, *Basic Works*. Ed. David Farrell Krell. New York: Harper & Row, 1977. 190–242.

Heidegger, Martin (1977) "The Question Concerning Technology." In *The Question Concerning Technology and Other Essays*. Trans. William Lovitt. New York: Garland Publishing. 3–35.

Houellebecq, Michel. (2024) Coronavirus: pour Michel Houellebecq, le monde d'après "sera le même, en un peu pire" (francetvinfo.fr). Accessed 1-16-2024.

Huebner, Sabine R (2021) "The 'Plague of Cyprian': A Revised View of the Origin and Spread of a 3rd-c. CE Pandemic," *Journal of Roman Archaeology* 34: 151–174.

Hugo, Victor (1874) *Quatrevingt-Treize*. Paris: Pocket, 1992.

Idema, Wilt L. (2021) *Sino-Platonic Papers* 313. https://medium.com/fairbank-center/plague-in-chinas-dynastic-twilight-faf6743ac8c1

Jablowska, Johanna (1993) *Literatur ohne Hoffnung: die Krise der Utopie in der deutschen Gegenwartsliteratur*. Wiesbaden: Deutscher Universitätsverlag.

Johansen, Bruce (1982) *Forgotten Founders: How the American Indian Helped Shape Democracy*. Boston: Harvard Common Press.

Jones, Reverend Penny. Julian of Norwich: 'all shall be well' (anglicanfocus.org.au). Accessed 3-14-2023.

Julian of Norwich (1675) *Revelations of Divine Love to Mother Juliana, Anchorite of Norwich*. Manuscript in British Library. Original 1675.

Kolb, Anjuli Fatima Raza (2021) *Epidemic Empire: Colonialism, Contagion, and Terror, 1817-2020*. Chicago: University of Chicago Press.

Judt, Tony (2001) "On 'The Plague,'" *New York Review of Books*. November 29. http://www.nyb00ks.com/articles/archives/2001/n0v/29/0n-the-plague/

Keller, Catherine (2018) *Political Theology of the Earth: Our Planetary Emergency and the Struggle for a New Public*. New York: Columbia University Press.

Keller, Catherine (2021) *Political Facing Apocalypse: Climate, Democracy, and Other Last Chances*. Maryknoll, NY: Orbis.

Kierkegaard, Søren (1941) *Alias Johannes De Silentio. Fear and Trembling: A Dialectical Lyric*, 1843. Trans. Walter Lowrie. Princeton: Princeton University Press.
Kufeld, Klaus. Ernst Bloch und das Prinzip Hoffnung. - YouTube.
Latour, Bruno (2015) *Face à Gaia: Huit conférences sur le nouveau régime climatique*. Paris: La Découvert. Trans. Catherine Porter as *Facing Gaia: Eight Lectures on the New Climatic Regime*. Cambridge, UK: Polity Press, 2017.
Latour, Bruno (2017) *Où atterrir? – Comment s'orienter en politique*. Paris: La Découverte. Trans. Catherine Porter as *Down to Earth: Politics in the New Climatic Change*. Cambridge, UK: Polity Press, 1988.
Latour, Bruno (2021) *Où suis-je? – Leçons du confinement à l'usage des terrestres*. Paris: La découverte. Trans. Julie Rose as *After Lockdown: A Metamorphosis*. Cambridge, UK: Polity Press, 2021.
Latour, Bruno (2001[1984]) *Pasteur: Guerre et paix des microbes*, suivi de *Irréductions*. Paris: La Découverte. Trans. A. Sheridan and J. Law as *The Pasteurization of France*. Cambridge: Harvard University Press, 1988.
Latour, Bruno (1996) *Petite réflexion sur le culte moderne des dieux faitiches*. Paris: La Découverte. First chapter trans. Catherine Porter and Heather MacLean as *On the Modern Cult of the Factish Gods*. Durham: Duke University Press, 2010.
Latour, Bruno (2022) *Qui perd la terre, perd son âme*. Paris: Balland. Trans. Catherine Porter and Sam Ferguson as *If We Lose the Earth We Lose our Souls*. Cambridge, UK: Polity, 2024.
Latour, Bruno and Peter Weibel, Eds. (2020) *Critical Zones: The Science and Politics of Landing on Earth*. Boston: ZKM and MIT Press.
Le Corguillé, Fabrice (2021) *Ancrages Amérindiens: Autobiographies des Indiens d'Amérique du Nord, XVIIIe-XIXe siècles*. Rennes: Presses Universitaires de Rennes. 1–20.
Levi, Primo (1989) *Se questo è un uomo*. Turin: Einaudi.
Li Shanbao (2021) *The Precious Scroll of the Rat Epidemic*. Trans. and Ed. Wilt L. Idema, *Sino-Platonic Papers* 313. Philadelphia: Department of East Asian Languages and Civilizations, University of Pennsylvania.
Löwy, Michael and Max Blechman (2008) "Négativité et espérance." In "T. W. Adorno-Ernst Bloch," Special Issue of Europe. SRevue *littéraire mensuelle* 86: 3–5.
Lovelock, James (2000 [1979]) *Gaia: A New Look at Life on Earth*. Oxford: Oxford University Press.
Lovelock, James (2006) *The Revenge of Gaia: Earth's Climate Crisis and the Fate of Humanity*. New York: Basic Book.
Luther, Martin (1552) "Ob man vor dem Sterben fliehen möge." In *Ausgewählte Schriften*, vol. 2, Ed. Hans Christian Knuth. Frankfurt am Main: Insel Verlag, 2016. Trans. Carl J. Schindler, "Whether One May Flee From a Deadly Plague" (1527). In *Luther's Works*, vol. 43, *Devotional Writings*. Ed. Gustav K. Wiencke. Philadelphia: Fortress Press, 1968.
Mallarmé, Stéphane (1945) *Oeuvres complètes*. Eds. Henri Mondor and G. Jean-Aubry. Paris: Pléiade.

Manigler, Patrice (2021) *Le philosophe, la terre et le virus: Bruno Latour expliqué par l'actualité*. Paris: Broché.
Manzoni, Alessandro (1985) *I promessi sposi*. Milan: Mondadori.
Manzoni, Alessandro (1993) *Storia della colonna infame*. Ed. Ferruccio Ulivi. Rome: Newton Compton.
Margulis, Lynn (1998) *Symbiotic Planet: A New Look at Evolution*. London: Weidenfeld & Nicolson.
McGrath, Sean L. (2021) *Thinking Nature: An Essay in Negative Ecology*. Edinburgh: Edinburgh University Press.
McLuhan, T. C., Ed. (1971). *Touch the Earth: A Self-Portrait of Indian Existence*. New York: Outerbridge & Lazaard. French Trans. *Pieds nus sur la terre sacrée*. Paris: Denoël, 2021.
McNeill, J. R. (2000) *Something New Under the Sun: An Environmental History of the Twentieth-Century World*. New York: W. W. Norton.
Meier, Franziska (2025) "The Witness: The use of the first-person narrative in the plague descriptions of Thucydides, Giovanni Boccaccio, Daniel Defoe, Alessandro Manzoni, and Albert Camus." *Narrating Pandemics: Transdisciplinary Approaches to Representations of Communicable Disease*. Ed. Andrew Gross, Silke Schicketanz and Richard Hoelzl. Toronto: University of Toronto Press.
Moltmann, Jürgen (1964) *Theologie der Hoffnung. Untersuchungen zur Begründung und zu den Konsequenzen einer christlichen Eschatologie*. Munich: Kaiser. Trans. Daniel L. Migliore as The Theology of Hope. New York: Harper & Row, 1967.
Moltmann, Jürgen (1985) *Gott in der Schöpfung: Ökologische Schöpfungslehre*. Gütersloh: Gütersloher Verlagshaus, 2015. Trans. *God in Creation*. London: SCM, 1985.
Moltmann, Jürgen (2019) "Theologie der Hoffnung im 21. Jahrhundert Vortrag von Prof. Dr. mult. em. Jürgen Moltmann Samstag, 3. August, Evangelische Akademie Bad Boll Im Rahmen der Blumhardt-Gedenk-Tagung 'Damit die Schöpfung vollendet werde.'" Available online at *Microsoft Word - Beitrag Moltmann (ev-akademie-boll.de). Accessed 3-17-2023.
Morgan, Thomas E. (1994) "Plague or Poetry? Thucydides on the Epidemic at Athens." *Transactions of the American Philological Association (1974-2014)* 124: 197–209.
Morton, Timothy (2007) *Ecology Without Nature*. Cambridge: Harvard University Press.
Morton, Timothy (2013) *Hyperobjects: Philosophy and Ecology after the End of the World*. Minneapolis: University of Minnesota Press.
Newheiser, David (2020) *Hope in a Secular Age: Deconstruction, Negative Theology, and the Future of Faith*. Cambridge: Cambridge University Press.
Nin, Anaïs (1969) *The Diary of Anaïs Nin*. Vol. 1, 1931–1934. Ed. Gunther Stuhlmann. Boston: Mariner Books.
Nothwehr, Dawn M. (2023) *Franciscan Writings: Hope amid Ecological Sin and Climate Emergency*. London: T&T Clark.

Pradeu, Thomas (2012) *The Limits of the Self: Immunology and Biological Identity*. Trans. Elizabeth Vitanza. Oxford: Oxford University Press.
Pradeu, Thomas (2020) *Philosophy of Immunology*. Cambridge: Cambridge University Press.
Primavesi, Anne (1991) *From Apocalypse to Genesis: Ecology, Feminism and Christianity*. Turnbridge Wells: Burns & Oates.
Primavesi, Anne (2000) *Sacrad Gaia*. London: Routledge.
Primavesi, Anne (2003) *Gaia's Gift: Earth, Ourselves and God After Copernicus*. London: Routledge.
Raffoul, François (2007) "Derrida et l'éthique de l'im-possible." *Revue de métaphysique et de morale* 53/1: 73–88.
Rey, Olivier (2018) *Leurre et malheur du transhumanisme*. Paris: Desclée de Brouwer.
Rey, Olivier (2020) *L'idolâtrie de la vie*. Paris: Gallimard.
Rosa, Hartmut (2018) *Unverfügbarkeit*. Frankfurt a.M.: Suhrkamp. Trans. James Wagner. *The Uncontrollability of the World*. New York: Polity, 2020.
Rose, Marika (2019) *A Theology of Failure: Žižek Against Christian Innocence*. New York: Fordham University Press.
Rosenzweig, Franz (S2002) *Der Stern der Erlösung*. Ed. Albert Raffelt. Freiburg im Breisgau: Universitätsbibliothek. Trans. William W. Hallo as *The Star of Redemption*. Boston: Beacon Press, 1964.
Ruether, Rosemary Radford (1992) *Gaia and God: An Ecofeminist Theology of Healing*. New York: HarperCollins.
Russell, Bertrand (1905) "On Denoting." *Mind* 14, no. 56: 479–493.
Scourfield, J. H. D. (1996) "The *De mortalitate* of Cyprian: Consolation and Context." *Vigiliae Christianae* 50: 12–41.
Shelley, Mary (1826) *The Last Man*. London: Colburn.
Smith, Anthony Paul (2003) *A Non-Philosophy of Nature: Ecologies of Thought*. London: Palgrave MacMillan.
Steenbuch, Johannes Aakjær (2022) *Negative Theology: A Short Introduction*. Eugene: Cascade.
Stengers, Isabelle (2009) *Aux temps des catastrophes: résister à la barbarie qui vient*. Paris: La Découverte.
Storm, Theodor (1863) "Märchen von der Regentrüde." *Leipziger illustrierte Zeitung*, July 30. In Theodor Storm, *Sämtliche Werke in vier Bänden*. Ed. Peter Goldhammer. Berlin: Aufbau, 1978.
Turner, Denys (1999) *The Darkness of God: Negativity in Western Mysticism*. Cambridge: Cambridge University Press.
Twain, Mark (1897) *Following the Equator: A Journey Around the World*. Hartford: American Publishing Company.
Valéry Paul (1919) *La Crise de l'esprit*. Paris: Éditions Robert Laffont, 405–414, 2000.
Vinale, Adriano (2020) "Epidemiologia politica: Foucault, Girard e la pandemia da Covid-19." *Storia e politica* 12/3: 416–436.
Vizenor, Gerald (1994) *Hiroshima Bugi: Atomu 57*. Lincoln: University of Nebraska Press.

Vizenor, Gerald (2003) *Manifest Manners: Postindian Warriors of Survivance*. Hannover: Wesleyen University Press.
Wald, Priscilla (2008) *Contagious: Cultures, Carriers, and the Outbreak Narrative*. Durham: Duke University Press.
Weber, Samuel (2022) *Preexisting Conditions: Recounting the Plague*. New York: Zone Books.
Wells, H. G. (1897) *The War of the Worlds*. London: Chapman and Hall.
West, David (2010) "Two Plagues: Virgil, *Georgics* 3.478-566 and Lucretius 6.1090-1286," *Creative Imitation and Latin Literature*. Eds. David West and Tony Woodman. Cambridge: Cambridge University Press.
White, Lynn (1967) "The Historical Roots of our Environmental Crisis." *Science* 155. Issue 3767. March 10: 1203–1207.
Wright, Lawrence (2020) *The End of October*. New York: Knopf.
Zakaria, Fareed (2020) *Ten Lessons for a Post-Pandemic World*. New York: Norton.
Žižek, Slavoj (2010) "A Meditation on Michelangelo's Christ on the Cross." In John Milbank and Slavoj Žižek, *Paul's New Moment: Continental Philosophy and the Future of Christian Theology*. Ed. Creston Davis. Grand Rapids: Brazos Press. 169–182.
Žižek, Slavoj (2020) *Pandemic: COVID-19 Shakes the World*. Cambridge: Polity Press.

Index

Abraham 115
Absolute 19, 20, 34
Adorno, Theodor 48
Agamben, Giorgio 40
All 50, 54, 55, 116; universal harmony of 81
Allegory 15
Apocalypse 17, 124; definition 44–45, 72; environmental 70–71; of Saint John 46, 123
Apophasis 53–54, 99
Arendt, Hannah 108
Aristotle 43
Artaud, Antonin 121, 133
Assman, Jan 95
Astrology 31
Axial Age 54–55
Augustine 13

Barrington Declaration 105
Barthes, Roland 37
Beauvoir, Simone de 37
Belonging vs. Liberation 96
Benjamin, Walter 33–34, 48
Bible 69, 101–103, 115; Creation story 102–103, 116; Exodus 127
Bloch, Ernst 4, 48–49
Bloomhardt, Christoph 101
Boccaccio, Giovanni 21, 26–27, 28–29, 36, 74, 131
Borromeo, Saint Carlo 30; Federigo 31

Buddhism 69
Butler, Judith 11, 41

Camus, Albert 15–16, 18–19, 36, 38–39, 122, 123, 133–134
Caputo, John 115
Cayley, David 104–105
China 55–59
Christianity 50, 96
Ciapelletto, Ser 25–26
Civil society 77–78
Climate change 71, 80
Colonial, language 2
Common 11
Conditionedness 38, 46, 97
Cone, James 50
Contingency 38
Control, compulsive 107–110
Cristoforo 31
Critical zone 89, 93
Cyprian of Carthage 117–118

Dante 123, 124, 126, 130–131
Daoism 3, 48, 69, 109
Death 9, 17, 73, 120; as absurd 18–19; and immortality 121
Defoe, Daniel 21, 27–28, 34, 107, 123, 132
Derrida, Jacques 16–17, 53, 113–114
Descartes, Renée 81
Desmet, Mattias 108
Destiny 36

Index

Dickinson, Emily xi
Don Quixote 60

Eagleton, Terry 49
Earth 4, 5, 79, 97; as one 94–95; its sovereignty 93; its transcendence 87–89, 94
Ecology 64–65, 69; dark 74; second-wave 75
Enlightenment 19, 31; its limits 39
Emancipation 96–97
Eschatology 93; ecological 97
Exodus 127

Failure 134
Faith 31
Fate 37
Fauci, Anthony 42
Faust 66–67, 69
Ferrante, Don 31
Fiction 20–21; self-critical 43–44
Folklore 14–15
Francis, Pope 63–67; on Dante as prophet of hope 131
Francis of Assisi xi; *Canticle to Brother Sun* 63–64, 81

Gaia 68, 70; transcendence of 89
God, hiddenness of 53; of many names 88; as Presence in Creation 77; transcends discourse 89; as unknowable 4, 41; wrath of 27, 46
Guardini, Romano 65
Guénoun, Denis 122
Guiscardo, Ruberto 124
Guttiérez, Gustavo 50

Hadot, Pierre 69
Harris, Sam 86
Heidegger, Martin 17, 49, 65–66, 85
Heraclitus 69
History, as revelation 20
Hölderlin, Friedrich 75
Homer, *Iliad* 15, 25, 73, 123, 127–128

Hope, definition of 50, 115; and helplessness 34, 38, 46, 122, 125, 133; principle of 49–50; and uncertainty 53
Horror films 134
Hugo, Victor 43
Humanism 15–16; critique of 17

Iamblichus 70
Idema, Wilt 56
Idolatry 40, 79–80, 87
Imagination 10, 45, 49; apocalyptic 28
Impossible 16, 115, 125–126
Incarnation 94
Indigenous 54, 77, 85; and emancipation 97; salvation 1–3, 4; studies 1; traditions 2
Infinity 11, 68–69
Information viral 113–114
Interconnectedness 11, 94–95

Julian, Emperor 69–70
Julian of Norwich 116–117, 122

Kafka, Franz 20, 36, 37
Kant, Immanuel 116
Keller, Catherine 46n10, 104
Kenosis 94
Kierkegaard, Søren 115
Kleist, Heinrich von 124
Kolb, Anjula Fatima Raza 37

Latour, Bruno 4, 79–80, 93–97; on science 83–84, 86; and theology 88
Lauterbach, Karl 42
Le Blanc, Judith 66
Levi, Primo 15, 109–110
Liberation 50, 96–97
Life 40–41
Literature 10
Lovelock, James 68, 70–71
Lucretius 25–26, 33, 128–129

Macron, Emanuel 41, 46, 80
Mallarmé, Stéphane 121–122

Manglier, Patrice 83
Manzoni, Alessandro 21–22, 30–32, 38–39, 74, 123, 132; *Infamous Column* 41–42
Marxist 49
Maxwell, William 44
McGrath, Sean 69, 100
Meier, Franziska 125
Metaphor 13
Merleau-Ponty, Maurice 11
Metaphysics 24
Milton, John 14
Moltmann, Jürgen 4, 48–50, 101–103, 104, 115
Morton, Timothy 74–75

Names, proper 89
Nature 69
Nazi 15, 109–110
Negative theology 48, 50, 88–89; and affirmative 20; constructive 4; definition of 3–4, 18; and horror films 134; and immanence 96; and kenosis 94; as negation of negation 68–69; thinks limits 93
Neoplatonism 69–70
New Climate Regime 80, 95–96
Nin, Anaïs 121
Non-identical 48
Non-resistance 58
Non-sovereignty 38
Normalcy 76, 106

Oedipus 14–15, 25
Openness 47; apophatic 54; and hope 122; to infinity 68–69
Original Sin 13–14, 131
Other 4, 18, 37, 38, 116; divine 40; suppression of 39
Ovid 33, 123, 130

Paul, Saint 13–14, 53, 97; on Creation 102; on hope 115
Plague, at Athens 25; and human limits 38–39; as incalculable 32; peters out 34–35; reconciles 107; as superhuman 36; as taboo 32; as unmasking 26; as within us 19, 133–134
Poe, Edgar Allan 132–133
Poetry 43, 129
Porter, Katherine Anne 43
Postmodern 12, 53
Primavesi, Anne 68–69
Progress 72–73
Psalms 28, 97–98

Rationalism 30; its limits 39
Rats 56–57
Real 18, 34; hyperreal 114; as whole 38, 45
Relatedness 4, 75–76; infinite 16; negative 43; self- 16; thinking 88; transformative 40; whole 58
Religion, new vs. cosmic 94–95; pagan 96; and science 97
Revelation, etymology 45; historical 20; non- 45, 93; through death 9; to ourselves 9, 119
Rey, Olivier 40–41
Ritual 70, 96, 100; burial 107
Romanticism 31, 52n3
Ruether, Rosemary 50
Russel, Letty 50

Salvation 94, 98; indigenous 99
Sartre, Jean-Paul 37
Scapegoat 41, 42
Scheler, Max 11
Science 82–84, 86; authority of 104–105; and religion 97
Self-critical 69, 116
Self-reflexivity 97
Self-sacrifice 31
Seneca 25, 128
September 11th (2001) 37
Shelley, Mary 52n3
Shi Daonan 56
Shoah 37
Smith, Adam 78
Smith, Anthony 69
Sophocles 128

Spanish flu 44, 72
Spengler, Oswald 49
Storytelling 34, 36
Supernatural 39
Survivance 3, 4, 57–58

Techno-science 38, 64–65
Technology 74–75; continuation of 97; critique of 85
Theology 44, 89; always negative 50, 88; of earth 101
Thinking 93, 100; contemplatively 99; negative 69; relational 88
Thucydides 25–26, 32–33, 74, 107, 125, 128–129
Time and eternity 95, 121
Tiresias 25
Totalitarianism 108
Transcendence 54; of divinity 50, 69–70, 85, 94; of Earth 87; and immanence 85, 87, 88; self- 86
Transhumanism 40, 73
Truth 84; personal 86; religious 88–89
Twain, Mark 43

Unknowability 4, 70
Unrepresentable 23
Unsayability 23, 37
Unthinkable 38, 44

Valéry, Paul 124
Virgil 33, 129–130
Vision, whole 10
Visionary 10, 39, 40, 72, 134
Vizenor, Gerald 3, 57–58
Vulnerability 4, 38, 58, 111; constitutive 19; insurmountable 17; and resilience 19

Wald, Priscilla 106, 113
War 39, 123–124; rhetoric 80
Weber, Samuel 10–11, 121, 122, 125; "frictional" 22–23
Wells, H. G. 36
Wet markets 71
Whole 10, 44, 58, 89, 111
World 47; end of 95, 120
Wright, Lawrence 12–13, 45, 111–112, 124, 134

Zakaria, Fareed 105
Žižek, Slavoj 11–12, 134

9781032895857